The Labour Ward Handbook

Benjamin
Black

D1337576

For
Orange Mummy

The Labour Ward Handbook

Second Edition

Leroy C Edozien

LLB BSc MSc MPhil MRCPI FRCOG FWACS
Consultant Obstetrician and Gynaecologist, St Mary's Hospital,
Manchester, UK; Honorary Senior Lecturer, Maternal and Fetal Health
Research Centre, The University of Manchester, Manchester, UK

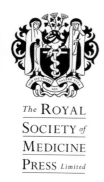

The ROYAL
SOCIETY *of*
MEDICINE
PRESS *Limited*

© 2010 Royal Society of Medicine Press Ltd

Published by the Royal Society of Medicine Press Ltd
1 Wimpole Street, London W1G 0AE, UK
Tel: +44 (0)20 7290 2921
Fax: +44 (0)20 7290 2929
E-mail: publishing@rsmpress.co.uk

British Library Cataloguing in Publication Data
A catalogue record for this book is available from the British Library

ISBN: 978-1-85315-810-0

Distribution in Europe and Rest of the World:
Marston Book Services Ltd
PO Box 269
Abingdon
Oxon OX14 4YN, UK
Tel: +44 (0)1235 465500
Fax: +44 (0)1235 465555
Email: direct.order@marston.co.uk

Distribution in USA and Canada:
Royal Society of Medicine Press Ltd
c/o BookMasters Inc
30 Amberwood Parkway
Ashland, OH 44805, USA
Tel: +1 800 247 6553/ +1 800 266 5564
Fax: +1 410 281 6883
Email: order@bookmasters.com

Distribution in Australia and New Zealand:
Elsevier Australia
30–52 Smidmore Street
Marrickville NSW 2204, Australia
Tel: +61 2 9517 8999
Fax: +61 2 9517 2249
Email: service@elsevier.com.au

Typeset by IMH(Cartrif), EH20 9DX, Scotland, UK
Printed in the UK by Bell & Bain, Glasgow, UK

Contents

Foreword

It is now six years since I wrote the foreword to the first edition of this handbook, and it is therefore timely that the guidelines it contains have been updated in a second edition. I suggested in the foreword to the first edition that knowledge is an organic, developing corpus, which, like plants, needs to grow and develop if it is not to wither. This is particularly true of guidelines, which shoud be nututred and maintained by regular review and evaluation. This is a huge task and we must be grateful that Leroy Edozien has undertaken it with energy, enthusiasm, diligence and skill.

The willing support of the publisher in bringing this second edition to fruition is a testament to the success of the first edition. There are many service directors who will be immensely grateful to Leroy for providing such a firm evidence-based foundation, from which their own locally appropriate guidelines can be developed and implemented. Tailoring is always necessary because of variations in local circumstances, but consistency is an important aspect of providing quality care to patients, as well as training to obstetricians and midwives. Migration from one unit to another on an annual basis has become mandatory in the training of obstetricians in the UK, and the turnover of midwifery staffing is often high, especially in urban areas where midwives commonly move to gain promotion. Regionalization of perinatal care is growing apace, emphasizing the need for consistency in management guidelines between different maternity units. It can be very confusing for patients and staff if transferral for tertiary care involves major changes in management strategy, particularly if changes are for reasons of local habit rather than being clinically necessary. National guidelines, for example, from the National Institute for Health and Clinical Excellence (www.nice.org.uk) in the UK, and from the National Guideline Clearinghouse (www.guideline.gov) in the USA, have grown substantially over the last six years, but the Internet is not always available, and it can be difficult to find the guidelines that one needs in any specific situation. Having a pocket-sized, handy summary of the key guidelines is a huge boon for the trainee and service director alike. Browsed frequently, it can help form the foundation of safe and effective clinical practice. This book now has secure roots and will, I am sure, continue to flourish for many years to come.

Professor Philip J Steer
Emeritus Professor in Obstetrics and Gynaecology,
Imperial College London

Preface

Clinical practice guidelines are here to stay. In high pressure situations such as the delivery suite, they can be invaluable. Unfortunately, many guidelines are written in the form of a textbook of theory and practice, not in a style that facilitates speedy reference. What busy staff *on the shop floor* need in the delivery suite is not a tome that describes underlying theories and research findings, but a handbook that succinctly spells out what should be done and when. *The Labour Ward Handbook* sets out to meet this need. The layout is reader-friendly, with less prose and more bullet points and tick boxes. References have been excluded from the main text and gathered at the end of each section under 'Further reading'. The tick boxes allow copies of the relevant pages to be inserted into the woman's hospital records, with the relevant boxes ticked, as a supplementary record of the woman's care during labour.

There are other principles which underpin this handbook. The first is a focus on the management of risk. Some of the chapters and the appendices specifically address risk issues, and other chapters have warning boxes or contain elements designed to help minimize human error. Secondly, although the chapters are mostly named after clinical conditions and processes, the woman is always at the centre of care – it is the woman rather than the condition that should be the focus. Thirdly, the book is addressed to both doctors and midwives, emphasising the team approach. Also, normal and abnormal labour are regarded as a continuum.

Clinical practice constantly changes as new evidence emerges, and every effort has been made to keep is second edition of *The Labour Ward Handbook* as up-to-date as possible. I hope that it will facilitate an evidence-based, but also holistic approach to care in labour.

LE

Acknowledgements

This book is a compendium of best practice distilled from a variety of sources, including research publications, textbooks, the Cochrane Library, guidelines produced by the UK National Institute for Clinical and Health Excellence (NICE) and by postgraduate medical colleges in the UK, Australia, Canada and USA, and the labour ward protocols of various hospitals, along with my own personal experience.

The book has its origins in guidelines that I compiled for the Royal Oldham Hospital ten years ago, with the support of the obstetric, midwifery, anaesthetic, paediatric and administrative staff of that hospital.

Dr Ross Macnab, Consultant Anaesthetist, Central Manchester University Hospitals Foundation Trust edited the chapters on epidural analgesia, recovery of the obstetric patient and high dependency care in both the first and second edition.

However, without the support of Peter Richardson, Managing Director of RSM Press, this book might not have been published, and the success of the first edition is a tribute to his foresight. My editors at RSM Press, Sarah McConalogue and Natalie Baderman for the current and previous editions respectively, have been very patient with me and have also produced attractive cover designs.

The contributions of all are acknowledged gratefully.

LE

Abbreviations

The following list includes those abbreviations used frequently in this book as well as those whose use is acceptable in written records (see p. 6):

ALT	alanine aminotransferase
APH	antepartum haemorrhage
APTT	activated partial thromboplastin time
ARDS	adult respiratory distress syndrome
ARM	artificial rupture of fetal membranes
bd	twice daily
BLS	basic life support
BP	blood pressure
CNST	Clinical Negligence Scheme for Trusts
CPR	cardiopulmonary resuscitation
CRP	C-reactive protein
CS	caesarean section
CSF	cerebrospinal fluid
CTG	cardiotocograph
CVP	central venous pressure
DDAVP	desmopressin acetate
DIC	disseminated intravascular coagulopathy
DVT	deep venous thrombosis
ECG	electrocardiography
ECV	external cephalic version
EUA	examination under anaesthetic
EWS	early warning score
FBC	full blood count
FBS	fetal blood sampling
FDP	fibrin degradation product
FFP	fresh frozen plasma
FH	fetal heart
FISH	fluorescence in situ hybridization
FSE	fetal scalp electrode
GBS	group B haemolytic streptococci
[Hb]	haemoglobin concentration
HDU	high-dependency unit
HELLP	haemolysis, elevated liver enzymes, low platelets
HIV	human immunodeficiency virus
HVS	high vaginal swab

IOL	induction of labour
IM (or im)	intramuscular
ITP	immune thrombocytopenic purpura
ITU	intensive therapy unit
IUGR	intrauterine growth restriction
IV (or iv)	intravenous
IVH	intraventricular haemorrhage
LFT	liver function tests
LMWH	low-molecular-weight heparin
MAP	mean arterial pressure
MRSA	Methicillin-resistant Staphylococcus aureus
NSAID	non-steroidal anti-inflammatory drug
NTD	neural tube defect
ODA	operating department assistant
OP	occipitoposterior
PDS	polydioxanone sulphate sutures
PPH	postpartum haemorrhage
PROM	prelabour rupture of fetal membranes
PT	prothrombin time
pv	per vaginum
qds	four times daily
RCM	Royal College of Midwives
RCOG	Royal College of Obstetricians and Gynaecologists
RDS	respiratory distress syndrome
Rh	rhesus
SBAR	situation, background, assessment, recommendation (a framework for effective communication)
SC (or sc)	subcutaneous
SCBU	special-care baby unit
SLF	systemic lupus erythematosus
SROM	spontaneous rupture of fetal membranes
ST	Specialty Trainee
tds	three times daily
TED	thromboembolism-deterrent stockings
U/E	urea and electrolytes
VE	vaginal examination
V/Q	ventilation–perfusion scan
VTE	venous thromboembolism
vWF	von Willebrand Factor

Glossary

Abnormal lie   Any lie other than longitudinal.

Advance decision   A declaration by a competent person stating what treatment should not be given if they lose the capacity to make decisions for themselves.

Anti-Xa assay   Test used to monitor heparin therapy. It measures the Xa inhibitory activity of heparin.

Arterial line   A cannula inserted into a peripheral artery (commonly the radial or brachial artery).

Bishop's score   A composite of five indices (station; position; consistency; effacement; and, dilation of the cervix), used to predict whether labour can be readily induced.

Central line   A catheter inserted into the superior vena cava or right atrium, usually via the right or left jugular or subclavian vein.

Central venous pressure (CVP)   Pressure in the superior vena cava or right atrium. This is used as a guide to fluid balance in critically ill women, and for monitoring circulatory collapse.

Chorionicity   The number of placentas in a multiple pregnancy – with a single shared placenta or one each.

Cleidotomy   Intentional fracture of the baby's collar bone, to facilitate delivery.

Clotting (or coagulation) profile   This usually comprises prothrombin time (PT), activated partial thromboplastin time (APTT), fibrinogen and fibrinogen degradation products (FDP).

D-dimer   A protein that is released into the circulation during the process of fibrin blood clot breakdown. D-dimer present in the circulation is used as an indicator of a blood clot being formed and broken down somewhere in the body. D-dimer levels in pregnancy are higher than in the non-pregnant state.

Dystocia   Dysfunctional labour.

Falx cerebri   A structure formed by two leaves of dura, along the sagittal suture.

Fifths palpable   The number of fifths of the baby's head palpable above the pelvic brim. This corresponds to the number of finger breadths palpable above the symphysis pubis. When the head is 'engaged', the bony presenting part (i.e. with the caput excluded) is at the level of the ischial spines, and the baby's head is 1/5 to 2/5 palpable abdominally.

Hydrops fetalis   A condition characterized by generalized oedema, often with ascites, pleural effusion and pericardial effusion.

Instrumental delivery   Vacuum-assisted (ventouse) or forceps delivery.

Ischial spines   A bony landmark in the pelvis; used to express the level of descent of the baby's head.

Malpresentation   Abnormal presentation – any presentation other than cephalic.

Operative vaginal delivery   Vaginal delivery by means of vacuum forceps.

Partogram   Graphic documentation of events in labour.

Patient group direction   A document that allows a registered healthcare professional (normally a nurse or midwife) to supply or administer a prescription-only medicine to a patient without the drug having been prescribed by a doctor.

Plasma substitute   Infusion used to expand and maintain blood volume. Gelofusine and Haemaccel are gelatine of bovine origin. They are recommended in this book since they have no effect on haemostasis. Maize starch products (e.g. Hespan) and hydrolysed starch (Dextran) inhibit clotting.

Rhesus isoimmunization   A condition arising from incompatibility of Rh blood groups in mother and baby.

Rule 42 (of the UKCC)   Midwives have a **statutory** duty to keep good records:

Rule 42(1):   'A practising midwife shall keep as contemporaneously as is reasonable detailed records of observations, care given and medicine or other forms of pain relief administered by her to all mothers and babies'.

Rule 42(3):   'A midwife must not destroy or arrange for the destruction of official records which have been made whilst she is in professional attendance upon a case ...'.

Tocolysis   Therapeutic arrest of uterine contractions.

Tocolytic   A drug used to stop uterine contractions.

Ventouse delivery   Vacuum-assisted delivery.

Bleep/crash calls

Bleeps

Obstetric ST (first on call) ......
Obstetric ST (second on call) ......
Paediatric ST (first on call) ......
Paediatric ST (second on call) ......
Anaesthetic ST ......
Anaesthetic assistant: ......

Emergencies

Crash calls for obstetric, paediatric and anaesthetic SpR

Obstetrics: ......
Ask for the appropriate doctor to be bleeped urgently. State the place (e.g. delivery suite and room number).

Paediatrics: ......
Request the second-on paediatrician urgently. State the place (e.g. delivery suite and room number).

Anaesthetics ......
State the place (e.g. delivery suite).

Note: If more than one of the specialties is required, it is not necessary to make more than one call. Bleep ...... and ask for an urgent call to go out to the appropriate specialties. State the place (e.g. delivery suite and room number).

Cardiac arrest ......
State the place (e.g. delivery suite and room number).

Fire
Activate the fire alarm. Dial ......

Wait for the call to be acknowledged. Proceed appropriately with the fire drill, as instructed at the annual fire lecture.

PART I
Approach to care

'... a shift in attention from what is done to patients to what is accomplished for them'

Committee on Quality of Healthcare in America. Institute of Medicine. Crossing the Quality Chasm: A New Health System for the 21st Century. Washington, DC: National Academy Press, 2001: 44

1 Communication

For efficient delivery of care, it is important that lines of communication are well defined. The consultant under whose care the mother is booked is ultimately responsible for her care. For each shift on the delivery suite, one midwife of appropriate seniority and experience will be designated Coordinator and will be responsible for coordinating the work of the delivery suite, providing necessary support, guidance and supervision of midwives and medical staff. The Coordinator should be informed regularly of each mother's progress. The names of the Coordinator and the obstetric, anaesthetic and paediatric medical staff on duty should be on the designated notice board.

The lines of communication for the midwife are through the Coordinator and the resident medical staff. However, any midwife or other member of staff who has concerns about a woman's care may contact the ST or consultant (obstetric or anaesthetic) directly.

All members of the duty obstetric team should ensure that they are readily accessible and available at all times.

Early identification and communication of risk

For women at high risk, a plan of management should be made antenatally and written in the handheld and hospital records, with a clear signature. Early identification of risk factors, anticipation of problems and effective communication are key factors for good management.

If a non-duty consultant has an interest in the management of a particular patient then this should be marked clearly in the case notes; the senior midwife or ST will need to contact this consultant when the woman is admitted and if problems arise afterwards.

All high-risk patients admitted to the labour ward must be seen by the doctor on duty as soon as possible.

The ST should be informed immediately of any untoward problems and of any of the following conditions (note that this is not an exhaustive list):

- APH
- PPH
- malpresentation
- cord prolapse/cord presentation

- severe pre-eclampsia/eclampsia
- multiple pregnancy
- preterm labour
- PROM
- abnormal fetal heart rate
- diabetes mellitus
- cardiac disease
- intrauterine death
- large baby
- previous CS
- any pregnancy identified as high-risk in the case notes

If there is any delay in response in cases such as prolapsed cord or if the registrar is unavailable because of another emergency, then the consultant on call should be called immediately.

It is recommended that the consultant should be physically present for the following:

- eclampsia
- maternal collapse (resulting from placental abruption, septic shock or other abnormality)
- CS for major placenta praevia
- PPH of more than 1.5 L where the haemorrhage is continuing and a massive obstetric haemorrhage protocol has been instigated
- return to theatre – laparotomy

Handover

There should be a personal handover of patient care at the shift/on-call changeover of both midwifery and medical staff. There should be ward rounds at 0830, 1300 and 1700 and a telephone review with the consultant at 2200.

There should be a professional approach to the ward rounds – which means no distractions such as telephone or side conversations. At each ward round, but particularly at the morning and evening rounds, there should be an assessment of the number and experience of the available workforce, identification of any threats to the service (e.g. non-availability of cots in the neonatal unit) and a review of patient safety incidents from the outgoing shift. The handover offers an opportunity to identify risks, make contingency plans and develop shared mental models for the challenges ahead. This helps to maintain situational awareness.

Communication with anaesthetists

In anticipation of events, the anaesthetist should be informed at an early stage of any of the following:

- APH
- twin pregnancy in labour
- breech vaginal delivery
- previous CS
- woman at risk of PPH
- pre-eclampsia
- obese patient who may require operative intervention
- medical conditions such as diabetes, sickle cell and heart disease
- history of anaphylaxis

'Anaesthetists responsible for obstetric services should liaise with midwives, obstetricians and physicians to agree management for successful delivery. The anaesthetist must become involved in the management of the "at risk" patient at an early stage ...'

Hibbard BM, Anderson MM, Drife JO, et al. *Report on Confidential Enquiries into Maternal Deaths in the United Kingdom 1991–1993.* London: HMSO, 1996: Chapter 9: 101

'Obstetricians failed to give adequate warning of impending problems to anaesthetic departments in at least six of the maternal deaths in this triennium. The lack of consultation with anaesthetic colleagues contributed significantly to a number of these deaths.'

Thomas TA, Cooper GM. Anaesthesia. In: Lewis G, ed. *Why Mothers Die, 1997–1999. The Fifth Report of the Confidential Enquiries into Maternal Deaths in the United Kingdom.* London: RCOG Press, 2001: 139

'A good working relationship between the multidisciplinary team (midwives, medical, ancillary, managerial staff) and the women in their care is crucial to ensure optimal birth outcomes. This is best achieved with a team approach, based on mutual respect, a shared philosophy of care and a clear organizational structure for both midwives and medical staff with explicit and transparent lines of communication. Clear, accurate and respectful communication between all team members and each discipline is essential, as well as with women and their families.'

Royal College of Obstetricians and Gynaecologists, Royal College of Midwives, Royal College of Anaesthetists, Royal College of Paediatrics and Child Health. *Safer Childbirth: Minimum Standards for the Organisation and Delivery of Care in Labour, Report of a Working Party.* London: RCOG Press, 2007: 10

2 Documentation

All records should be written in black ink, and handwriting must be legible. The care given should be documented carefully and thoughtfully. All examinations, results, clinical communications and maternal requests should be documented accurately on the labour notes, partogram and CTG trace as appropriate.

All entries to the records must be clearly signed, dated and timed (use the 24-hour clock). Illegible signatures are not acceptable. Always print your name and grade below your signature.

Use abbreviations sparingly, and only those in standard use (eg CS, FH).

Every loose-leaf sheet in the notes must have patient identification. The responsibility for this rests with the first person who writes on that page.

Consent for examination, CS and other interventions must follow standard policy and practice (see Appendix 1).

Every operative delivery should be written up in detail, with the date, time, indication(s), findings and any complications stated clearly. Instructions for postoperative care should be itemized. Proformas for CS, instrumental vaginal delivery and repair of perineal tears help to raise the quality of documentation.

The time of decision to perform a CS, and the degree of urgency (see p. 82), should be documented. The time of commencement of CS, i.e. 'knife to skin', should be recorded in the theatre log book.

Before filing any results, check that they belong to the correct patient, annotate any action required or taken, and append your signature.

Every CTG trace should bear the patient's identification label and the date and time of commencement and completion. The maternal pulse should be recorded regularly on the trace (not just at the beginning), along with any key events in care. Any loss of contact or discontinuation should be annotated on the trace.

Sign and date all CTGs, and file them securely with the clinical records.

The standard setting of 1 cm/min should not be altered on the CTG monitor.

Never try to alter existing notes. If corrections are necessary, draw a line through the incorrect entry and sign and date the additional note.

All midwifery records must comply with standards set by the Nursing and Midwifery Council (see Further reading, p. 16).

The statutory limitation on obstetric litigation is not until the child is 21 years of age, so notes relating to pregnancy care must be maintained intact for this duration.

3 Admission to, and discharge home from, the delivery suite

Admission

The initial assessment will be by a named midwife to whom the woman has been introduced. Where indicated (see Chapter 1), the admitting midwife should refer to the doctor on duty, without delay. The antenatal clinic records and records of any admissions in the pregnancy should be reviewed and any special instructions noted. A plan of care should be devised with the woman, building on wishes and plans agreed during antenatal care. This plan should be flexible, and subject to review during labour. Document the reason for admission, the findings on assessment and the plan of care.

Discharge

An experienced midwife may discharge a woman home when labour has been excluded, provided that the following criteria are met:

- ☐ normal, uneventful pregnancy at 37–40 weeks
- ☐ normal medical history
- ☐ normal maternal observations
- ☐ normal/reactive admission CTG, where this test is indicated
- ☐ no abnormal vaginal loss
- ☐ normal vaginal examination with no indication that labour has established
- ☐ intact membranes
- ☐ first referral to delivery suite
- ☐ woman is happy to go home
- ☐ follow-up appointment is given

A woman who presents with deviations from the above criteria should be referred to the doctor on call for further assessment. A woman not wishing to go home may be transferred to the antenatal ward.

4 Learning from clinical incidents

The labour ward should have formal systems for learning from clinical incidents and for sharing lessons learned. Apart from structures and processes such as the multidisciplinary labour ward forum and mechanisms for reporting incidents, a culture of safety has to be nurtured.

What is a clinical incident?

A clinical incident (also known as a patient safety incident, adverse event, or critical incident) is an untoward event that happened to a woman during or as a result of care or treatment and that has caused, or could cause, an adverse outcome.

All incidents on the trigger list, and any others that, in the opinion of the ward manager, fall within the scope of this definition, must be reported as detailed below.

It is not practicable to provide an exhaustive list of clinical incidents, but the more common examples are:

- maternal death
- stillbirth
- neonatal death
- low Apgar score: <6 at 5 minutes
- undiagnosed breech
- shoulder dystocia
- major PPH (≥1000 mL)
- postpartum [Hb] < 8 g/dL
- eclampsia or other fits
- unexpected transfer to neonatal unit, including neonatal seizures
- medication errors
- significant infections
- loss of clinical materials (e.g. swabs)
- unavailability of health record
- return to theatre
- third- and fourth-degree tears
- readmission of either mother or baby
- unavailability of any facility or equipment, including neonatal unit cots
- misdiagnosis of antenatal screening tests

- unplanned home birth
- cord pH < 7.05
- maternal transfer to ITU
- maternal resuscitation
- injury to bladder or other organs
- first stage of labour >17 hours
- second stage of labour >3 hours
- birth injury
    - subdural haematoma or tear of falx cerebri
    - any fracture (e.g. skull, clavicle, long bone)
    - any paralysis (e.g. brachial plexus injury)
- low cord pH
- major congenital abnormalities first detected at delivery
- any event considered to be serious, regardless of outcome

Why do we need clinical incident analysis?

By continual review of clinical incidents, we could improve care and reduce risks to women:

- Near-misses are an important source of information to prevent such events happening again.
- Identification of common themes can help to predict and prevent future incidents.
- Early warning signs can be picked up.

We can promote a culture of learning and enquiry, and help all members of the multidisciplinary team to reflect on their practice and make changes as necessary. The principle is not to blame or shame, but to promote active learning and improve the quality of care.

Clinical incidents are commonly due to inadequacies in the system rather than the fault of an individual. Analysis of incidents will be used to determine how the system can be improved, and not to punish the individual. The analysis will be used to identify unexpected events and those with poor outcomes that may need further investigation. Once risk factors or patterns emerge, we can focus on prevention and education. Information could alert line managers to possible weaknesses in systems of work.

Clinical incident analysis will provide an archive of facts for possible use in medico-legal cases.

Reporting clinical incidents

Incidents should be reported using the hospital's incident-reporting form (electronic or paper) and in line with the hospital's risk management strategy.

Learning from clinical incidents

In addition to use of the incident reporting system, the unit will identify clinical incidents and risks through prospective risk assessments, clinical audit, complaints and claims. Reported incidents will be analysed and investigated as stipulated in the hospital's risk management strategy. Periodic summaries of reported incidents will be provided. It is more important to report what changes have been implemented and what demonstrable benefits have resulted from reported incidents.

Lessons learned from the identification and treatment of risk should be shared with other parts of the hospital/trust and with the wider community as may be appropriate, through channels such as multidisciplinary team meetings, ward meetings, safety alerts, newsletters, intranet and educational meetings.

The labour ward/maternity unit should have a risk register that lists major risks and what control measures are in place or planned. A maternity 'dashboard' is also a useful device for monitoring progress with risk control.

Confidentiality

Practitioners are expected to respect the confidentiality of their patients and colleagues when undertaking a review. Information will be handled at all times in a way that protects patients' confidentiality, and in keeping with the Data Protection Act. Anonymous reporting is preferable to concealment. Incidents or near-misses may be reported anonymously or (preferably) confidentially to the ward manager, the consultant or the risk management midwife.

5 Transfer of care between professionals

Background

This guidance stems from recommendations by various bodies concerned with quality of care:

- The NHS Litigation Authority (NHSLA) standards call for clear arrangements concerning which professional is responsible for the patient's care at all times.
- The *Confidential Enquiries into Stillbirths and Deaths in Infancy (CESDI)* emphasized the importance of adequate arrangements for transfer of patients between units.
- The Royal Colleges, in the document *Towards Safer Childbirth*, state that explicit lines of communication between professionals are crucial to optimization of birth outcomes.

Handover by clinical staff

There should be a formal handover on the ward at 0830, 1300 and 1700 on weekdays and at 0900 at weekends. The handover takes priority over other, non-emergency clinical duties.

The baton bleep should be handed over personally to the incoming person – it is unacceptable to leave the bleep at the ward station or reception.

Transitions of care between individual practitioners and between clinical areas should follow a formal local protocol. The outgoing practitioner should summarize in writing the clinical status of the woman (including the Early Warning Score (EWS), where applicable) and itemize what needs to be done. The SBAR (Situation, Background, Assessment, Recommendation) framework is recommended for communicating transfers of care.

Transfer of emergencies from primary care

Emergency transfers to the labour ward can be made at any time by the GP or community midwife after discussion with the medical or midwifery staff. The coordinator must be informed. Some referrals will be more appropriate to the maternity day assessment unit or the early pregnancy assessment unit, and should be directed accordingly.

Transfer between hospitals with the fetus in utero

- ☐ All transfers in or out must be with the prior approval of the consultant obstetrician.
- ☐ If there is a good chance that the baby will need to be delivered in the next 48 hours then availability of a cot in the neonatal unit of the receiving hospital must be confirmed before transfer.
- ☐ Where indicated, prophylactic steroids should be given before transfer in or out.
- ☐ Where indicated, a tocolytic should be given before transfer in or out.
- ☐ Appropriate personnel should accompany the woman. The coordinating midwife and the consultant obstetrician will determine the appropriate personnel for each case.
- ☐ Do not transfer (or accept a transfer) if any of the following apply:
  - uncontrolled vaginal bleeding
  - cervix >4 cm dilated
  - three or more uterine contractions in 10 minutes.
- ☐ A letter and a copy (not the original) of the notes should accompany the woman.
- ☐ Results of relevant investigations should be recorded in the notes or telephoned through to the receiving hospital as soon as they are available.
- ☐ For women transferred from another hospital, an MRSA screen should be performed on admission

Transfer of care between consultants

When a patient is referred to a special or subspecialty clinic, there should be a referral letter indicating whether this is an outright transfer or a request for opinion only.

For emergency admission of unbooked patients, the woman is under the consultant on call at the time of admission, unless she has an unfinished clinical episode under another consultant, in which case she remains under that consultant's care. A clinical episode, in this context, finishes when a discharge letter has been written.

Transfer back to the community or GP care

Follow-up plans/arrangements should always be specified in the case notes (hospital and handheld) and in discharge letters. If no follow-up appointment has been arranged then this should be stated in a discharge letter.

Following a stillbirth, miscarriage or termination for fetal anomaly, the GP, community midwife and health visitor must be informed immediately (see also pp. 235–236).

Where it has been arranged for a patient to be followed up by the community midwife, this should be documented in the case notes and in the diary kept on the unit.

Transfer to ITU and HDU

Who transfers?

A patient may be transferred to ITU or HDU at the request of the consultant obstetrician/gynaecologist, consultant anaesthetist or anaesthetic registrar. All transfers to ITU must be discussed first with the consultant anaesthetist in charge.

Who is in charge while the woman is in ITU or HDU?

A patient in ITU is primarily under the care of the consultant anaesthetist, but the consultant obstetrician remains responsible for the obstetric care. Any woman admitted into ITU must be seen daily by the obstetric team.

The consultant obstetrician/gynaecologist is primarily responsible for the care of his or her patient transferred to the HDU.

Return to delivery suite from ITU

The consultant obstetrician and consultant obstetric anaesthetist should be involved in the decision to transfer/accept the transfer from ITU to delivery suite, and one of them should see the woman before she is transferred. The SBAR framework is recommended for a structured transfer.

Both the physical and the psychological needs of the woman should be addressed.

If possible, transfers from the ITU to the delivery suite at night should be avoided.

6 Reviewing what happened

It is often helpful if the newly delivered mother has an opportunity to discuss her experience with a professional who was involved in her care. Events are reviewed and, where necessary, issues are clarified.

The review provides the opportunity for the mother to:

- ask questions
- express her feelings, e.g. pleasure, gratitude, fear, anger, confusion or other emotions
- understand the reasons for unmet expectations
- be reassured of her success and her achievement
- be given explanations and apologies, as may be necessary
- plan for future pregnancies

The review should be held at a mutually convenient time before discharge. The format of the review is not prescriptive. It should be a listening and sharing activity, not a counselling activity.

A summary of the following should be recorded in the postnatal records:

- ☐ date and time of meeting, and who attended
- ☐ matters discussed
- ☐ questions asked
- ☐ unresolved issues, if any
- ☐ further action required

Where difficulties are experienced, support and advice should be sought from a ward manager, supervisor or consultant or from the hospital's patient advice and liaison service.

Some women may prefer to speak with a midwife or obstetrician who was not involved in the delivery.

If a complaint is imminent then the hospital's complaints policy should be followed.

Further reading for Part I

Communication

NHS Litigation Authority. *Clinical Negligence Scheme for Trusts: Maternity Clinical Risk Management Standards*. Version 2, 2009/10. London: NHS Litigation Authority, April 2009.

Royal College of Obstetricians and Gynaecologists, Royal College of Midwives, Royal College of Anaesthetists, Royal College of Paediatrics and Child Health. *Standards for Maternity Care. Report of a Working Party*. London: RCOG Press, 2008. Available at: www.rcog.org.uk/womens-health/clinical-guidance/standards -maternity-care.

Royal College of Obstetricians and Gynaecologists, Royal College of Midwives, Royal College of Anaesthetists, Royal College of Paediatrics and Child Health. *Safer Childbirth: Minimum Standards for the Organisation and Delivery of Care in Labour. Report of a Working Party*. London: RCOG Press, 2007. Available at: www. rcog.org.uk/files/rcog-corp/uploaded-files/WPRSaferChildbirthReport2007.pdf.

Royal College of Obstetricians and Gynaecologists. *Responsibility of Consultant On-Call*. Good Practice No. 8. London: RCOG, March 2009. Available at: www.rcog. org.uk/responsibility-of-consultant-on-call.

Documentation

Cowan J. Clinical governance and clinical documentation: still a long way to go? *Clin Perform Qual Health Care* 2000; **8**: 179–82.

NHS Litigation Authority. *Clinical Negligence Scheme for Trusts: Maternity Clinical Risk Management Standards*. Version 2, 2009/10, April 2009.

Nursing and Midwifery Council. *Midwives Rules and Standards*: Rule 9 – Records, August 2004. Available at: www.nmc-uk.org/aDisplayDocument. aspx?documentID=169.

Nursing and Midwifery Council. *Record Keeping*. Advice Sheet, July 2009. Available at: www.nmc-uk.org/aDisplayDocument.aspx?DocumentID=6269.

Clinical incident reporting

Department of Health. *An Organisation with a Memory. Report of an Expert Group on Learning from Adverse Events in the NHS*. London: The Stationary Office, 2000.

Royal College of Obstetricians and Gynaecologists. *Improving Patient Safety: Risk Management for Maternity and Gynaecology*. Clinical Governance Advice No. 2. London: RCOG, 2005. Available at: www.rcog.org.uk/improving-patient-safety-risk-management-maternity-and-gynaecology.

Royal College of Obstetricians and Gynaecologists. *Maternity Dashboard Clinical Performance and Governance Score Card*. Good Practice No. 7, London: RCOG, January 2008. Available at: www.rcog.org.uk/files/rcog-corp/uploaded-files/ GoodPractice7MaternityDashboard2008.pdf.

PART II
Normal and low-risk labour

'I have stated on numerous occasions that there is no more need to interfere with the course of normally progressing labor than there is to tamper with good digestion, normal respiration, and adequate circulation'.

Montgomery TL. 1958 Physiologic considerations in labor and the puerperium. *Am J Obstet Gynecol* 1958; **76**: 706–15

7 Vaginal examination

Before vaginal examination

☐ Consent must be obtained.
☐ The history should be reviewed.
☐ Ultrasound scan results should be noted, where applicable.
☐ Abdominal examination and auscultation should be performed.

During vaginal examination

• Ensure privacy and dignity.
• Communicate with the woman.
• Be alert to non-verbal cues. This is particularly important for women with past traumatic experiences.

Details to be recorded

☐ Date and time
☐ Findings on abdominal examination
☐ Indication for vaginal examination
☐ Relevant information on condition of external genitalia and vagina
☐ Cervical effacement (the length of the cervical canal in centimetres)
☐ Cervical dilatation
☐ Presentation:
    • level of presenting part in relation to ischial spines
    • application to cervix
    • caput
    • moulding:
        +   skull bones apposed
        ++   reducible overlap of bones
        +++ irreducible overlap of bones
☐ Membranes:
    • intact or absent
    • colour and volume of amniotic fluid
☐ Fetal heart auscultation following procedure
☐ Findings explained to mother
☐ Signature and printed name

8 Intravenous cannulation

Intravenous cannulation is recommended for patients with:

- previous PPH
- grandmultiparity (fifth and subsequent labours)
- anaemia ([Hb] < 10 g/dL)
- multiple pregnancy
- previous CS (undergoing a trial of vaginal delivery)
- meconium-stained amniotic fluid
- high-risk pregnancy, where the likelihood of operative intervention or peripartum haemorrhage is significant

10 mL of blood for group-and-save serum and FBC should be sent to the laboratory. All group-and-save serum samples should be signed by two professionals.

The cannula should be flushed using either 5 mL 0.9% saline or 5 mL (50 iu) heparin sodium.

Syntocinon (oxytocin) infusion may be commenced as per patient group direction when:

- induction of labour has been agreed previously by an obstetrician
- there is slow progress and the obstetrician on call has confirmed that labour should be augmented

All indications, discussions and agreement should be documented.

In the event of PPH occurring, an infusion of 40 units Syntocinon in 500 mL Hartmann's solution may be commenced while awaiting medical assistance.

No IV fluids other than those indicated on the patient group direction should be given without being prescribed by a doctor.

9 Management of normal labour

Normal labour will be managed by the midwifery staff. A comprehensive risk assessment should be undertaken when a woman is admitted in labour, and risk is continually assessed during labour.

Criteria for normal labour

Normal labour is defined by the presence of all of the following criteria:

- [ ] uncomplicated pregnancy (most women will have been booked for midwifery-led care)
- [ ] spontaneous onset of labour at 37–41 weeks' gestation
- [ ] minimum rate of cervical dilation 1 cm/h from diagnosis of established labour
- [ ] first admission to labour ward
- [ ] single fetus with engaged head
- [ ] clear amniotic fluid
- [ ] normal maternal observations
- [ ] no intrapartum bleeding
- [ ] no maternal or fetal distress
- [ ] normal delivery within 1 hour of good expulsive effort
- [ ] intact perineum, first- or second-degree tear or episiotomy
- [ ] third stage lasts for less than 20 minutes following active management
- [ ] immediate postpartum blood loss < 500 mL

The doctor should be called to see any woman falling outside these criteria.

Initial assessment on admission should include the following:

- [ ] BP
- [ ] pulse rate
- [ ] respiratory rate
- [ ] temperature
- [ ] urinalysis
- [ ] recording of the fetal heart with a handheld Doppler device
- [ ] abdominal palpation: symphysio–fundal height, presentation, position and fifths palpable (see Glossary)

- ☐ uterine contractions: frequency, duration and strength
- ☐ fetal membranes and, if they are ruptured, colour of amniotic fluid (clear/blood-stained/meconium-stained)
- ☐ MRSA assessment, if indicated and as directed by local policy

10 Prelabour rupture of membranes at term (37–42 weeks)

A woman with suspected spontaneous rupture of membranes and no associated contractions or vaginal bleeding may be assessed (CTG, sterile speculum examination) on the antenatal ward, in the day unit or at triage.

If the woman is bleeding or has uterine contractions then she should be admitted to the delivery suite. If the CTG is abnormal, the woman must be seen immediately by a doctor.

An experienced midwife may perform a speculum examination provided that the following criteria are met:

- normal uneventful pregnancy at 37–40 weeks
- normal fetal heart rate
- no vaginal bleeding
- consent obtained

If there are no uterine contractions it is not necessary to perform a digital examination.

A vaginal swab should not be taken as a routine, but the clinician can use their judgement to decide when a vaginal swab might give clinically useful information.

If PROM is confirmed, the woman should be advised that:

- the risk of serious neonatal infection is 1 in 100 (compared with 1 in 200 for women with intact membranes)
- 6 of every 10 women with PROM at term will go into labour within 24 hours
- induction of labour is appropriate approximately 24 hours after rupture of the membranes

The mother may be observed on the antenatal ward if PROM is confirmed and the following criteria are met:

- no meconium-stained amniotic fluid
- cephalic presentation, well-applied to the cervix
- normal maternal observations
- <24 hours have elapsed since rupture of the membranes

If any of these criteria do not apply then the obstetrician on call should be informed.

Where PROM is excluded, the discharge protocol should be followed.

Further management

Women with confirmed PROM should be offered a choice of expectant management (not exceeding 72 hours) or immediate induction of labour.

The benefits and risks of expectant management versus immediate induction of labour should be discussed, and the agreed plan should be documented. A Cochrane review detected no differences with regard to mode of birth between immediate induction of labour and expectant management – the concern that immediate induction might result in more caesarean and operative births was not supported. Significantly fewer women in the planned management group compared with the expectant management group had chorioamnionitis or endometritis. No difference was seen in terms of neonatal infection, but fewer infants under planned management went to neonatal intensive or special care compared with expectant management.

If the woman is known to be group B haemolytic streptococcus-positive, labour should be induced immediately and antibiotics should be prescribed (see pp. 210).

Expectant management

Await spontaneous onset of labour.

Antibiotics

Antibiotics should not be given in the absence of signs of infection. If there are signs of infection then prescribe a full course of broad-spectrum IV antibiotics.

When to intervene

If there are any clinical signs suggestive of infection (tachycardia, pyrexia), induce labour.

If observations are normal but labour does not ensue, induce after 12–72 hours (as agreed with the woman).

Induction protocol (see p. 100 for details)

- Bishop score < 5: prostaglandin 1 mg (or 2 mg if nulliparous). Reassess 6 hours later if not in labour.
- Bishop score ≥ 5: Syntocinon infusion.

Observe the baby

When 18 hours have elapsed since rupture of the membranes, antibiotics should be given (see pp. 207).

If labour has not started 24 hours after PROM, the woman should be advised to stay in hospital for at least 12 hours following the birth – so that the baby can be observed for signs of infection. The baby, if asymptomatic, should be observed at 1 hour, 2 hours and then 2-hourly for 10 hours. These observations should include:

- general wellbeing
- chest movements and nasal flare
- skin colour, including perfusion, by testing capillary refill
- feeding
- muscle tone
- temperature
- heart rate and respiration

Active management

Induce with prostaglandin or Syntocinon, as above. See p. 99–103 for the protocol for induction of labour.

An alternative, but unlicensed, option is active management with oral or vaginal misoprostol:

- oral 50 mg, repeated every 4 hours if required, to a maximum of five doses
- vaginal 25 μg (50 μg in nulliparous women with Bishop score ≤ 4), followed by 25 μg after 4 and 8 hours

In an Aberdeen study, 9 out of 10 women on the oral regimen were in labour within 24 hours. Uterine rupture following induction of labour with misoprostol has been reported, and the dose stated above should not be exceeded. The sublingual route of administration is as effective as the vaginal route in inducing labour in full-term pregnancies, but its safety has not been established.

Dose

Ranitidine 150 mg orally every 6 hours until completion of the third stage. Women who are vomiting, who have had opioid analgesia or who are otherwise unable to take oral medication should be given ranitidine 50 mg IM 6-hourly.

Women not in labour but undergoing a 'crash' CS should have IV ranitidine 50 mg in 20 mL 0.9% saline over 2 minutes and IV metoclopramide 10 mg. See also p. 83.

Pain relief

The woman should be informed of the various methods of pain relief that are available. The analgesia requested should be administered and documented as per patient group direction.

Breathing, relaxation and massage techniques may be used.

Transcutaneous electrical nerve stimulation (TENS) should not be offered to women in established labour.

Entonox (50% O_2 and 50% N_2O)

Fully disposable breathing systems should be used. Where this is not available, the Entonox apparatus should include anti-infective filters.

The woman should be informed that it may make her feel nauseous and light-headed.

Opioids (pethidine, diamorphine or other)

The woman should be informed of the side-effects: drowsiness, nausea and vomiting in the mother; short-term respiratory depression and drowsiness in the baby.

Pethidine

In established labour, pethidine may be given, in a dose dependent on the woman's weight:

<60 kg 100 mg IM 3–4-hourly
>60 kg 150 mg IM 3–4-hourly

An antiemetic (e.g. metoclopramide 10 mg IM) should be given with the first dose of pethidine.

Diamorphine

Compared with pethidine, this is associated with a higher level of pain relief, less maternal vomiting and a lower incidence of low 1-minute Apgar scores.

Epidural analgesia

Women offered epidural analgesia should be informed of the risks and benefits, and the implications for their labour.

See p. 42 for the care of a woman who wishes to have epidural analgesia.

Bladder care

Over-distension of the bladder could cause denervation and permanent damage to the bladder. Encourage the woman to empty her bladder at least every 3 hours, and document the volume passed. If she is unable to void urine after 4 hours, inform the doctor.

If an indwelling catheter is needed for any reason, use the smallest size possible, to reduce irritation of the urethra.

Vaginal delivery should not be conducted with a catheter still in place, since this could injure the urethra.

12 Fetal monitoring

A risk assessment is done on admission to the delivery suite. For low-risk women, the fetal heart may be auscultated intermittently using a fetal stethoscope (Pinard) or Doppler ultrasound (Sonicaid). See pp. 3–4 for a list of some conditions that exclude women from this group.

For at-risk women, a CTG is mandatory on admission. Continuous electronic monitoring is required in the following situations:

- epidural sited
- Syntocinon infusion in progress
- fresh meconium-stained amniotic fluid
- high-risk pregnancy (maternal or fetal problems)
- maternal request
- intermittent auscultation reveals decelerations
- baseline fetal heart rate <110 or >160 beats/min
- vaginal bleeding
- maternal pyrexia

> **!** Before commencing CTG or intermittent auscultation, palpate the maternal pulse simultaneously with auscultation to differentiate between maternal and fetal heart tones.

Intermittent auscultation

Auscultate for 60 seconds, beginning immediately after the end of a contraction, every 15 minutes in the first stage of labour and every 5 minutes in the second stage.

Electronic fetal monitoring

- ☐ Check that the date and time clocks on the monitor are set correctly.
- ☐ Ensure that the paper speed is set to 1 cm/min.
- ☐ Label the paper with the woman's identifying details.
- ☐ If a good trace cannot be obtained using an abdominal transducer then use a scalp electrode. If the signal is still poor then the presence of fetal heart pulsation should be confirmed by an ultrasound scan.

FSE is contraindicated in:

- women with HIV or hepatitis virus
- fetal bleeding disorders (e.g. haemophilia)

Suspicious or abnormal trace

If any fetal heart rate abnormality is identified then monitoring should be continuous and, where necessary, an FSE should be applied. The coordinating midwife should be informed; if she/he is not happy then the doctor on call should be asked to review.

Any midwife or doctor reviewing a trace should document on both the trace and the case notes, stating their findings and plan.

When describing and acting on a CTG, the following features should be documented:

- ☐ frequency and strength of uterine contractions
- ☐ baseline fetal heart rate
- ☐ variability
- ☐ presence or absence of accelerations
- ☐ presence or absence of decelerations
- ☐ overall assessment and plan, taking into account any background risk

Every woman in labour having electronic fetal monitoring should have the trace reviewed at least every hour using the classification below.

Classification of cardiotocograph (Table 12.1)

- **Normal:** all four features of the cardiograph are normal.
- **Suspicious:** one feature is non-reassuring.
- **Pathological:** two features are non-reassuring, or there is at least one abnormal feature.

Management of suspicious or pathological cardiotocograph

- ☐ The patient should be in the left lateral position.
- ☐ Inform the registrar.
- ☐ Exclude hypotension; give crystalloid infusion if appropriate.
- ☐ Exclude hypercontractility; stop Syntocinon infusion.
- ☐ Check maternal pulse and temperature.
- ☐ Exclude cord prolapse (vaginal examination).

Table 12.1 Classification of cardiotocograph

Classification	Baseline (beats/min)	Variability	Deceleration	Acceleration
Reassuring	110–160	≥5	None	Present
Non-reassuring	100–109, 161–180	<5 for 40–90 min	Early deceleration Variable deceleration Deceleration for ≤3 min	
Abnormal	<100, >180 Sinusoidal pattern for ≥10 min	<5 for ≥90 min	Late deceleration Atypical variable deceleration Prolonged deceleration for >3 min	

☐ If the trace is pathological or persistently suspicious then FBS is indicated (see Chapter 13).

Do not give oxygen to the mother, since it may be harmful to the hypoxic baby

Management of fetal tachycardia

Ask the following questions:

• Is there an obvious explanation?
• How severe is the tachycardia?
• Are there other complications (decelerations, loss of variability) on the CTG?
• Is delivery imminent?

Take the following action:

☐ Check maternal pulse and temperature.
☐ Correct dehydration.
☐ If the fetal heart rate is 160–180 beats/min and the trace is uncomplicated then no intervention is required.
☐ If the tachycardia is persistent and >180 beats/min then do FBS. If FBS is not feasible then discuss with the consultant and proceed to CS.

Note

In cases of fetal sepsis, there could be tachycardia with normal fetal scalp blood pH. Bear this in mind where there has been prolonged rupture of fetal membranes.

Management of fetal bradycardia

Assess the following:

- depth of bradycardia
- duration of bradycardia
- signs of recovery (rapid or slow?)
- variability
- nature of the trace prior to bradycardia
- if in second stage, is delivery imminent?

Take the following action:

- ☐ Adopt left lateral tilt.
- ☐ Turn off Syntocinon infusion.
- ☐ Check and record maternal pulse.
- ☐ Check BP.
- ☐ If the woman is hypotensive or has just had an epidural, give a rapid infusion of IV fluid. (*Note*: following an epidural, a drop in fetal heart rate may occur even with a normal BP.)
- ☐ Perform a vaginal examination to exclude cord prolapse and to assess cervix and descent.
- ☐ If there is vaginal bleeding then consider the possibility of placental abruption or uterine rupture.
- ☐ If there is no recovery by 6 minutes, prepare for operative delivery (CS or instrumental).

Scalp pH should not be performed for prolonged bradycardia.

> **!** If there is bradycardia lasting up to 10 minutes then proceed straight to CS (or instrumental delivery if feasible).

Schedule

- **1–5 minutes**: call for help. Review as outlined above.
- **6 minutes**: expect recovery towards baseline. If there is no recovery then prepare for operative delivery.

- **9 minutes**: if there is no recovery, transfer to theatre (or effect instrumental delivery if feasible).
- **15 minutes**: baby delivered.

Reduced variability (2–5 beats/min)

- This may reflect fetal sleep.
- Has the mother had a narcotic drug or sedation?
- If it lasts longer than 40 minutes then do FBS (or discuss with consultant if FBS is not feasible).

Absent variability (<2 beats/min) calls for immediate intervention.

When interpreting a complicated CTG, pay particular attention to the variability.

A more accurate picture of variability is obtained from a scalp electrode than from an abdominal transducer. The latter tends to overestimate variability.

Late deceleration

Take the following action:

- ☐ Adopt left lateral tilt.
- ☐ Turn off Syntocinon infusion.
- ☐ Check BP.
- ☐ Perform a vaginal examination to exclude cord prolapse and to assess cervix and descent.
- ☐ If the cervix is ≥3 cm dilated then do FBS. If it is <3 cm dilated then proceed to CS.

Decelerations in the second stage of labour may be innocent or indicative of hypoxia.

Assess the following:

- nature of trace in the first stage of labour
- depth, duration and recovery of decelerations
- variability

If these give cause for concern then operative delivery is indicated (see also 'Contraindications to fetal blood sampling' in Chapter 13).

13 Fetal scalp blood sampling

If the CTG is suggestive of fetal distress then FBS from the scalp should always be undertaken before proceeding to CS, unless it is technically not possible to do so.

☐ Explain the procedure to the woman and obtain consent.
☐ The cervix must be at least 3 cm dilated and the presenting part should be no more than 2 cm above the plane of the ischial spines.
☐ The patient should be in the left lateral position or in the lithotomy position with a wedge.
☐ At least two samples should be taken on each occasion. After obtaining each sample, ensure haemostasis by applying pressure with a swab on the stab site.
☐ Inform the patient of the result and plan.

Contraindications to FBS
- prolonged (>10 minutes) fetal bradycardia
- pathological CTG associated with APH, suspected chorio-amnionitis, or possible rupture of uterine scar
- pregnancy <34 weeks
- full cervical dilatation and presenting part below spines – **deliver the baby!**
- HIV-positive or hepatitis B-positive/C-positive mother; active herpes
- fetal bleeding disorder (e.g. haemophilia)

Interpretation of pH result
Normal values
- pH >7.25
- pO_2 > 2.6 kPa (> 20 mmHg) (note that pO_2 is not of value in assessing risk to the baby)
- pCO_2 < 8 kPa (< 50 mmHg)
- base excess > 8 mmol/L

Results should be interpreted in the context of clinical features, rate of progress in labour and previous pH reading:

- ≥7.25: normal; may need repeating if CTG abnormality persists. If the FBS result is stable after the second test then, provided that there are no additional abnormalities on the trace, a third test may be deferred.

- **≤7.20:** acidosis; delivery indicated.
- **7.21–7.24:** repeat within 30 minutes, or consider delivery if there has been a rapid fall since the last sample.

If two neat samples were obtained, management should be based on the lower pH. If no good sample was obtained, FBS should be repeated – do not derive false reassurance from an inadequate sample.

Scalp blood lactate

This is an alternative to pH measurement, and is done using commercially available test strips. Anaerobic metabolism produces lactate, so levels of this metabolite are a measure of tissue hypoxia. Measurement of lactate in fetal scalp blood requires a much smaller volume of blood and its predictive value for fetal acidosis is similar to that of pH measurement. It is not in widespread use in the UK.

Documentation

- ☐ Obtain verbal consent.
- ☐ The pH meter printout, labelled and dated, should be secured with sticky tape in the case notes.
- ☐ Document the plan of management following blood sampling.

FBS at full cervical dilatation

If the cervix is fully dilated and the presenting part is below the plane of the ischial spines then the woman should be offered instrumental delivery.

If the presenting part is still high, FBS may be performed. A normal result allows time for descent of the presenting part, thus allowing a normal delivery or increasing the chances of a successful instrumental delivery.

> **!** If FBS has been performed then cord-blood sampling must be performed at delivery.

14 Augmentation of labour

If labour is slow then consider the following possible causes:

- prolonged latent phase of labour (safe to augment)
- inefficient uterine activity (generally safe to augment)
- obstructed labour (dangerous to augment)

Artificial rupture of fetal membranes (ARM)

> 'The older doctrine of the sanctity of the membranes was more or less built in with the bricks in my obstetrical philosophy. No labour is so pleasing and satisfactory to mother and child as when intact membranes are maintained right up to full dilatation at which point a gush of clear, clean liquor amnii flushes out the genital tract, followed, not so many minutes later, by the delivery of a clean, healthy, screaming baby. This is Nature at her best and I never cease to marvel at such normality'.
>
> Donald I. *Practical Obstetric Problems*, 5th edn.
> London: Lloyd-Luke, 1979: 566

ARM should not be performed routinely, but it may be used to accelerate labour if progress is slow (<1 cm/h). It should be discussed with the woman before the vaginal examination is performed.

The rate of progress must be considered in the context of the mother's circumstances. A rate of 1 cm/h in a woman who is having strong uterine contractions and who is in severe distress is more worrying than a rate of 0.5 cm/h in a woman who is comfortable and mobile.

The midwife may rupture the membranes artificially (for induction or augmentation of labour) if the following criteria are met and the mother consents:

- [ ] The head is engaged.
- [ ] The vertex is presenting.
- [ ] Cord presentation has been excluded.

Contraindications to ARM are:

- abnormal lie
- cord presentation
- placenta praevia

After ARM, check for cord prolapse and meconium staining of amniotic fluid. Document the fetal heart rate.

Augmentation with Syntocinon

Syntocinon (oxytocin) may be prescribed to accelerate labour, provided that the following conditions are met:

- ☐ Presentation is cephalic.
- ☐ Membranes have ruptured.
- ☐ Amniotic fluid is clear.

Syntocinon infusion should not be started until 6 hours have elapsed since administration of prostaglandin.

Syntocinon should not be used in secondary arrest (after 5 cm dilatation) until obstructed labour has been excluded by vaginal examination. Particular care should be taken in multiparous women.

The use of Syntocinon in the following circumstances requires the explicit approval of the consultant:

- multiple pregnancy
- malpresentation
- previous CS or other uterine scar
- grandmultiparity

If augmentation of labour is indicated then the midwife, per patient group direction, may commence an IV infusion of Syntocinon:

- if maternal and fetal wellbeing are normal
- following discussion with obstetrician on call
- with documentation in labour records

When labour is augmented with Syntocinon, a vaginal examination should be performed 4 hours after commencing the infusion. If there is less than 2 cm progress after 4 hours of Syntocinon then CS should be considered.

Syntocinon infusion

Mix 10 units of Syntocinon in 500 mL Hartmann's solution. Commence infusion at 2 milliunits/min (i.e. 6 mL/h). Increase every 30 minutes until strong, regular uterine contractions – three in 10 minutes – are obtained.

A syringe driver or infusion pump must be used.

Do not exceed 32 milliunits/min (i.e. 96 mL/h); see Table 14.1.

Do not infuse through the same line as blood, plasma or insulin.

The syringe must be labelled, with the dose of drug and signatures of responsible staff on the label.

All women for whom labour is being augmented with Syntocinon should have continuous electronic fetal monitoring.

Second stage of labour

Syntocinon infusion may be given to augment uterine contractions in the second stage of labour, providing that obstructed labour has been excluded by abdominal and vaginal examination.

Mix 10 units of Syntocinon in 500 mL Hartmann's solution. Commence infusion at 2 milliunits/min (i.e. 6 mL/h). Increase every 15 minutes until strong, regular uterine contractions – three in 10 minutes – are obtained.

Uterine hyperstimulation

Manifestation

- More than five contractions per 10-minute interval for at least 20 minutes (uterine tachysystole), or each uterine contraction lasting up to 2 minutes or increased baseline uterine tone (uterine hypertonus).
- Suspicious or pathological CTG.

Table 14.1 Regimen for Syntocinon infusion

Time after starting (min)	Rate (milliunits/min)	Rate (mL/h)
0	2	6
30	4	12
60	8	24
90	12	36
120	16	48
150	20	60
180	24	72
210	28	84
240	32	96

Management

- Discontinue Syntocinon infusion.
- Lay the woman on her left side.
- Institute a rapid infusion of 1000 mL 0.9% saline.
- In extreme cases, consider tocolysis with terbutaline 0.25 mg SC. *Note:* This is an off-licence use of terbutaline.
- It may be necessary to deliver the baby – is the CTG back to normal?

15 Cord-blood sampling

Blood should be obtained for acid–base status from an isolated segment of umbilical cord following delivery of any potentially acidotic fetus, including:

- intrapartum CTG
- cases where fetal scalp blood has been sampled
- instrumental vaginal delivery
- preterm delivery
- breech vaginal delivery
- IUGR
- placental abruption
- cord prolapse
- baby born with a low Apgar score
- fetal abnormality

A quality control check must be made on the analyzer as directed by the manufacturer (see the handbook accompanying the machine).

A 10 cm segment of cord is clamped immediately after delivery of the baby.

Samples of cord artery and vein are obtained with pre-heparinized syringes. The arterial sample is more difficult to obtain, but this is the sample that is representative of the baby's acid–base balance. Unless both arterial and venous samples are obtained, it cannot be established that the umbilical artery has been sampled.

The segment of cord (or the sample in the pre-heparinized syringe) may be left at room temperature for up to 30 minutes (or in ice for up to 1 hour) before analysis.

Inform the duty paediatrician if the arterial pH < 7.05 or if the venous pH < 7.20.

! Beware – with some analyzers, the quality control printout could be mistaken for the actual specimen result.

16 Epidural analgesia in labour

Epidural analgesia in labour requires a resident anaesthetist and continuous care and monitoring of the mother and fetus by a suitably trained midwife. If either is unavailable then epidural analgesia should not be instituted. Patient information about epidurals and other forms of pain relief should be available.

The woman should be informed that epidural analgesia is associated with a longer second stage of labour and an increased chance of vaginal instrumental birth, but is not associated with long-term backache or with a longer first stage of labour or an increased chance of caesarean birth. If the epidural solution contains opioids, the mother should be informed of the risk of short-term respiratory depression and drowsiness in the baby.

Indications for epidural analgesia

- maternal request
- occipitoposterior position
- induced/accelerated labour
- prolonged labour
- multiple pregnancy
- breech presentation
- pre-eclampsia (see below)
- premature birth/high-risk fetus
- maternal medical problems (e.g. diabetes, asthma and certain cardiac problems)

Contraindications to epidural analgesia

- maternal refusal
- coagulopathy (see below)
- shock/uncorrected hypovolaemia
- inadequate staffing
- septicaemia
- local infection
- raised intracranial pressure
- allergy to amide local anaesthetics (rare)

Coagulopathy

The risks and benefits of epidural analgesia/anaesthesia need to be assessed in each case. It is not possible to lay down absolute criteria. A regional block is usually given if the platelet count is above 100×10^9/L, but epidural analgesia may be withheld if the count is higher than this but falling rapidly. A coagulation profile must be done if the platelet count is <100×10^9/L, and a senior anaesthetist must be involved.

A platelet count should be done in the case of pre-eclampsia and where there has previously been a low count.

In addition, PT, APTT and FDPs should be checked in the following cases:

- severe pre-eclampsia (including HELLP)
- intrauterine death
- placental abruption

Therapeutic/prophylactic anticoagulation

See also pp. 172 and 179.

Some women will have had LMWH – usually dalteparin (Fragmin) – for prophylaxis or treatment of thrombosis. This is not an absolute contraindication to regional block.

Peak anti-Xa activity (see Glossary) is reached about 3 hours after a subcutaneous injection of LMWH, but 50% of peak levels are still present at 12 hours. Spinal/epidural should be inserted at least 12 hours after a prophylactic dose and 24 hours after a therapeutic dose. Patients on any anticoagulant should have PT and APTT checked before placing an epidural/spinal, but note that these are unlikely to be affected by LMWH.

Setting up

Exact equipment requirements vary between anaesthetists. The following are usually required:

- ☐ IV cannula (minimum 16G, i.e. grey Venflon) with a 1000 mL bag of Hartmann's solution connected via a blood-giving set
- ☐ epidural trolley, fully stocked (the stock list is on the trolley)
- ☐ resuscitation equipment, including oxygen and suction
- ☐ patient's records and an epidural chart
- ☐ BP and fetal heart monitoring equipment
- ☐ tilting bed
- ☐ wedge

The anaesthetist will want to know:

- parity
- whether there has been a previous epidural
- stage and progress of labour
- other analgesia used
- significant obstetric and medical problems
- maternal BP and vaginal examination findings

Procedure

☐ The procedure is explained by the anaesthetist. Verbal consent is obtained and documented.

☐ Ask the woman to empty her bladder.

☐ A preload of IV fluid may be given but is not routinely required before establishing low-dose epidural analgesia and combined spinal–epidural analgesia. The drip must be able to flow freely if needed.

☐ The woman should be either on her side or sitting on the side of the bed and leaning over a table.

☐ An appropriate area of the back (L2–3 or L3–4) should be cleaned with chlorhexidine spray.

☐ The midwife should support the mother during the procedure, particularly with regard to maintaining good position.

☐ After catheter insertion, a test dose of local anaesthetic is given to exclude placement in the cerebrospinal fluid or a vein.

☐ BP and pulse rate should be checked every 5 minutes for a further 15–20 minutes, during which time the mother should not be left unattended.

Method of administration

When the epidural catheter has been inserted, continuous analgesia can be administered by one of the following means:

- infusion
- boluses (top-ups)
- controlled epidural analgesia
- spinal epidural

Epidural infusion

Continuous infusion reduces, but does not eliminate, the need for bolus injections. Often at least one top-up is required. There are two reasons for this:

- Epidural drug requirements tend to increase as labour progresses.
- Infusion rates sufficient to eliminate the need for top-ups often cause excessive blocks and are therefore best avoided.

The anaesthetist will prescribe a low-dose anaesthetic agent (e.g. 10–15 mL of 0.0625–0.1% bupivacaine with 1–2 micrograms/mL fentanyl) and the infusion rate. When indicated, the infusion rate should be adjusted as outlined in Table 16.1.

High concentrations of local anaesthetic solutions (≥0.25% of bupivacaine or equivalent) should not be used routinely for either establishing or maintaining epidural analgesia.

The following observations are required hourly:

- ☐ volume infused
- ☐ infusion rate
- ☐ presence or absence of excessive motor block (inability to bend both knees)
- ☐ block height (test for cold sensation or pinch in the epigastrium; sensation should be normal here)

Inform the anaesthetist if:

- pain does not respond to a top-up after 20 minutes
- abnormal epigastric sensation persists 30 minutes after reducing the infusion rate
- excessive motor block persists 30 minutes after reducing the infusion rate

Table 16.1 Adjustments to infusion rate when there is a problem

Finding	Action
Mother in pain	Administer top-up (see p. 46) and increase rate by 2 mL/h
Epigastric cold/pinch	Reduce rate by 2 mL/h
Sensation abnormal	Recheck in 30 min
Excessive motor block	Reduce rate by 2 mL/h Recheck in 30 min

Epidural top-up

A trained midwife may give top-ups of anaesthetic in doses prescribed by the anaesthetist. The anaesthetist must be available within 5 minutes if there are problems. Typical doses are 10–15 mL 0.125% bupivacaine or 15 mL of 0.1% bupivacaine with 2 µg/mL fentanyl, given every hour.

Protocol for top-ups

☐   A top-up is indicated if the mother is in pain and feels that her analgesia is inadequate.

☐   Check epidural prescription (**do not rely on oral instructions**).

☐   Check maternal pulse and BP, motor block and block height. Contact the anaesthetist if there are any adverse findings.

☐   Check bladder fullness and empty as necessary.

☐   Draw up the prescribed dose of anaesthetic agent. **This must be checked with a second midwife**.

☐   Do not administer epidural drugs during a contraction.

☐   The mother should be in a sitting or full lateral position.

☐   Administer the drug in a divided dose.

☐   The initial fraction must be given *slowly*. Over the next 5 minutes, observe/ask about any sudden increase in motor block, dizziness, tingling in the face and tinnitus.

☐   At 5 minutes, check maternal pulse and BP. **The upper arm will under-read BP if the patient is in a lateral position**. If dizziness, tingling or another symptom is observed or if the systolic BP falls below 90 mmHg (or by >30 mmHg) then omit the remaining fraction and call the anaesthetist. Otherwise, administer the remaining dose and continue observing for these symptoms or hypotension.

☐   Check BP every 5 minutes for a further 15–20 minutes. The woman must not be left unattended during this time.

> **!** If the top-up is ineffective after 20 minutes, call the anaesthetist.

If hypotension occurs at any stage, treat as outlined under 'Hypotension' on p. 48 and call the anaesthetist.

General care of the woman with an epidural

The woman should be looked after by a dedicated and suitably trained midwife. The anaesthetist remains responsible for the regional block and should attend regularly, not just when called by the midwife.

If the midwife has any concerns about the epidural (see 'Complications' below) then the anaesthetist should be contacted.

The woman should be encouraged to move and adopt whatever upright positions she finds comfortable throughout labour. She should never be supine. If she is on her back, then a wedge must be under the right buttock at all times, even during vaginal examination. At other times, the sitting position is preferred. If the woman wishes to lie down then the full lateral position is acceptable.

- ☐ Hourly position changes (to avoid pressure-related problems) should be continued until the epidural has worn off completely and should be recorded on the appropriate chart.
- ☐ Maternal BP should be checked every 30 minutes.
- ☐ There should be continuous fetal heart monitoring (note that CTG abnormalities may occur up to 1 hour after an epidural).
- ☐ Temperature should be checked every 4 hours.
- ☐ Encourage bladder emptying every 2 hours and before top-ups. Palpate regularly to detect urinary retention. Record urine output.
- ☐ Perform vaginal examination as indicated (with wedge in place).

In the second stage of labour

- Breakthrough pain may occur. A top-up should be offered. This should be given in the sitting position to block the sacral root.
- The epidural infusion should not be stopped. If the woman is totally unaware of her contractions (which is not common in practice) then she should be encouraged to push when contractions are palpated. The prescribed infusion rate may be reduced by 2 mL/h in these circumstances. There is insufficient evidence to suggest that stopping an epidural late in labour lowers the risk of instrumental delivery or other unwanted outcomes.
- In the second stage of labour, unless the woman has an urge to push or the baby's head is visible, pushing should be delayed for at least 1 hour – longer if the woman wishes – after which pushing during contractions should be actively encouraged.
- Perineal infiltration may still be required before episiotomy.

Complications of epidural analgesia

Inadequate analgesia

- This may occur at some stage in up to 20% of epidurals.
- Give a top-up as detailed above and call the anaesthetist if this is ineffective after 20 minutes.

Hypotension

Prevention

☐ Make the appropriate checks before giving a bolus.
☐ The woman should avoid the supine position at all times.
☐ Correct any pre-existing hypovolaemia.

If the systolic BP falls below 90 mmHg (on the lower arm if the woman is in the lateral position):

☐ Turn the woman to the full lateral position. If this is ineffective, then:
☐ Fully open the drip and give 500 mL compound sodium lactate (Hartmann's solution).
☐ Give oxygen by facemask (minimum 10 L flow with wall oxygen).
☐ Call the anaesthetist.
☐ Have ready a box of ephedrine, water for dilution and a 10 mL syringe.

Dural tap

- This occurs when the epidural needle or catheter accidentally penetrates the dura, usually resulting in a leak of cerebrospinal fluid.
- Immediate management varies between cases. The anaesthetist will leave specific instructions.
- Any further bolus doses of local anaesthetic must be administered by the anaesthetist.
- **There is no evidence to support elective instrumental delivery**.
- The patient should be informed of the puncture.
- Inform the anaesthetist if the woman develops a headache.

Local anaesthetic toxicity (IV injection)

Suspect this if the epidural catheter is blood-stained and the epidural not effective. Features include tinnitus, tingling in the face, dizziness, confusion, slurred speech, loss of consciousness and cardiovascular collapse. If the woman has any of these during a bolus, stop the injection and call the anaesthetist. Turn the woman to the lateral position, give oxygen and check her vital signs.

Total spinal

This occurs when the catheter is placed intrathecally.

The features are rapid onset of analgesia and a dense motor block, followed by nausea and vomiting, pallor, and sweating, possibly leading to loss of consciousness and apnoea (cessation of breathing).

BP will be very low. Maternal heart rate may be high or low. The fetal heart will almost certainly deteriorate.

Initial treatment is as for hypotension:

- Place the woman in the full lateral position.
- Open the drip fully.
- Give oxygen by mask (this may need the support of breathing; check breathing and commence basic life support if needed).
- Call the anaesthetist.
- Have ephedrine and a cardiac arrest trolley ready in the room.

Dense motor block

The woman should not mobilize until motor block has worn off. The block has worn off when the woman is able to straight-leg raise, bring her knees up to her chest, and push hard against resistance with both feet, without difficulty in both lower limbs.

There should be hourly position changes, to prevent pressure-related problems. These should be continued until the motor block has worn off completely.

Bladder distension

Regular voiding should be encouraged during labour, particularly before a bolus is given and until the epidural has worn off. Distension may be palpable and/or may cause breakthrough pain. In-and-out catheterization should be performed if the woman is unable to void spontaneously.

! Call the anaesthetist if any of the following occur:
- inadequate anaesthesia
- hypotension
- headache following dural tap
- symptoms of local anaesthetic toxicity (see previous page)
- dense motor block
- any other concern

Discontinuation of epidural

- After delivery, remove the catheter with a gentle, steady pull, ideally with the woman in the same position as during insertion. The tip of the catheter should be checked for completeness and a record made.
- Before removing the catheter, always check whether LMWH was given. If LMWH was given, at least 12 hours must elapse before the catheter is removed.
- The woman should not be allowed to mobilize until she is able to flex both hips and knees against resistance. She should be accompanied when she first walks.

17 Management of the second stage of labour

The second stage of labour comprises:

(a) **passive second stage:** the cervix is fully dilated but there are no involuntary expulsive contractions
(b) **active second stage:** the cervix is fully dilated, there are involuntary expulsive contractions and the baby is visible

Once the second stage has been diagnosed, the woman should not be left without a midwife in attendance. Essential elements of care commenced in the first stage of labour – such as psychological support and hydration – should be continued in the second stage.

The woman should be encouraged to give birth in the position that she finds most comfortable. The recumbent position tends to lengthen labour, to reduce the incidence of spontaneous birth and to increase the incidence of abnormal fetal heart rate patterns.

Regardless of whether it is a normal delivery or an instrumental delivery, only the accoucheur and no more than one assistant should be at the lower end of the woman's body.

Fetal heart rate should be recorded at least after every second contraction. BP should be recorded half-hourly if normal, but every 15 minutes in hypertensive women.

> **!** Always be certain that the cervix is fully dilated.

Duration

There is no evidence to suggest that the imposition of an upper time limit for the duration of the second stage improves the outcome for mother or baby. More important than the time factor are evidence of progressive descent and maternal and fetal wellbeing.

Passive phase

Labour that is progressing normally may be in the passive stage for 1 hour. In a woman who has not had epidural analgesia, if the vertex is not visible within the hour then a vaginal examination should be performed.

Active phase

The doctor should be informed if the baby has not been delivered after 2 hours of pushing in a nullipara or after 1 hour in a multipara.

Immediate versus delayed pushing

A nulliparous woman with epidural analgesia may start pushing within an hour of full cervical dilatation (immediate pushing) or after up to 2 hours in the passive phase (delayed pushing). A meta-analysis of seven random-allocation trials showed that delayed pushing (passive descent) was associated with an increased chance of spontaneous vaginal births, a decreased risk of instrumental delivery and a shorter pushing time.

Encourage active pushing when:

- the woman has a desire to push and the vertex is visible on gently parting the labia
- 1 hour has elapsed since full dilatation was confirmed, and the presenting part is below the plane of the ischial spines

Observations and assessment in second stage:

- ☐ Take BP and pulse hourly.
- ☐ Take temperature 4-hourly (continued from first stage).
- ☐ Document frequency of contractions at least half-hourly.
- ☐ Empty the bladder.
- ☐ Perform a vaginal examination after 60 minutes of pushing or where there is concern (e.g. cord prolapse).
- ☐ Measure fetal heart rate. If using intermittent auscultation, do this every 5 minutes.

Steady progress should be made in the active stage. Keep the coordinating midwife informed. Progress must be assessed by abdominal as well as vaginal examination (see p. 26).

Delayed second stage

Inform the doctor if:

- after 1 hour in the passive phase, the presenting part is not visible
- a nulliparous woman is undelivered after 2 hours of active pushing
- a multiparous woman is undelivered after 1 hour of active pushing

Management

☐ Exclude disproportion. Excessive caput and moulding are indicative of obstruction.

☐ If contractions are inadequate and there are no contra-indications, commence Syntocinon (oxytocin) infusion. Contraindications include disproportion, abnormal CTG and possible rupture of scar.

☐ Evaluate for instrumental delivery (see p. 90)

A situation to be avoided:

'In the second stage it is common to see assistants crowding at the lower end of the woman's body, anxiously watching her vulva as if waiting for luggage to appear in an airport carousel.'

Sheila Kitzinger. Birth and violence against women –
generating hypotheses from women's accounts
of unhappiness after childbirth.
In: Roberts H, ed. *Women's Health Matters*.
London: Routledge, 1992: Chap 4

Calling the paediatrician

In some cases, it will be necessary to call the paediatrician in the second stage of labour, when delivery is imminent – see Chapter 18. It is advisable to document the time when this call is made.

18 Criteria for paediatric attendance at delivery

If any of the following are noted, a paediatrician should be called to attend the delivery:

- fetal distress
- abnormal presentation
- prolapsed cord
- APH
- meconium-stained amniotic fluid
- forceps/vacuum-assisted delivery (except lift-out procedures, where there is no fetal distress)
- CS if performed under general anaesthesia or if there is a fetal indication (e.g. IUGR)
- severe pre-eclampsia
- drug abuse/addiction by mother
- diabetes mellitus
- multiple pregnancy
- breech vaginal delivery
- preterm delivery (<36 weeks)
- Rh isoimmunization
- fetal hydrops
- polyhydramnios
- congenital abnormalities
- anticipated shoulder dystocia
- concern of attending midwife/obstetrician

In the case of prolonged rupture of membranes (>24 hours), ear and umbilical swabs should be obtained from the baby and the paediatrician should be informed.

> **!** The midwife or obstetrician should use their clinical judgement to determine whether to call the first on-call or second on-call paediatrician, depending on the degree of risk.

19 Management of the third stage of labour

Active management of the third stage of labour significantly reduces the risk of PPH, regardless of the posture of the mother or the experience of the midwife, but there is a slight increase in the incidence of nausea and vomiting.

Active management is the recommended practice unless the mother makes an informed choice to have physiological management. The mother's choice should be documented clearly on her birth plan and labour record.

A combination of active and physiological management is unacceptable.

Physiological management is contraindicated in the following circumstances:

• operative delivery
• induced or augmented labour
• polyhydramnios
• previous PPH
• epidural analgesia
• diabetes mellitus
• prolonged labour
• multiple pregnancy
• APH
• anticoagulant therapy
• anaemia
• grandmultiparity

Active management

(1) Give an oxytocic drug with delivery of the anterior shoulder. IM Syntometrine (ergometrine with oxytocin) 1 mL to the upper thigh muscle is the drug of choice unless contraindicated, in which case give IM Syntocinon (oxytocin) 10 IU.

   Contraindications to Syntometrine:
   • hypertension, pre-eclampsia
   • severe cardiac disease
   • pulmonary oedema
   • hepatic or renal impairment

(2) Clamp the cord early (within 1–3 minutes of birth).

(3) Deliver the placenta and membranes by controlled cord traction with the next uterine contraction.

If the woman has not delivered within 30 minutes, refer to the obstetrician.

Physiological management

- Do not give any oxytocic drug.
- Leave the cord to pulsate; do not clamp or cut.
- Adopt careful watching and waiting. Do not apply any cord traction.
- Encourage breastfeeding.
- Observe for signs of separation: lengthening of cord, gush of blood or rise of the uterine fundus.
- Encourage maternal effort aided by gravity.
- **If the woman has not delivered within 1 hour (earlier if there is concern regarding blood loss or maternal condition) then refer to the obstetrician.**

20 Immediate postpartum care

It is advisable for the mother and baby to remain in the midwife's care, on the delivery suite, for 1 hour after delivery. If there are any deviations from normal wellbeing of the mother or the infant then the obstetrician or paediatrician must agree transfer to the postnatal ward.

The drug chart should be checked before transfer to the ward to ensure that analgesics, antibiotics, thromboembolism prophylaxis and other medication have been prescribed as required.

Care of the mother

The mother's general wellbeing, pulse, BP and temperature should be recorded. Assessment of uterine retraction and vaginal blood loss should also be documented. The mother should be offered a bed bath or shower, as well as light refreshment, and made comfortable before arrangements for her transfer to the postnatal ward.

If an epidural catheter is in place then it should be removed before the mother leaves the delivery suite. The tip of the catheter should be checked for completeness and a record made (see p. 50).

Bladder care

Over-distension of the bladder could cause denervation and permanent damage to the bladder. Ensure that the woman has voided urine prior to leaving the delivery suite, and document the time and volume of the first void. If she has not voided, inform the staff on the postnatal ward. If a woman has not voided urine 6 hours post delivery, a catheter should be introduced. A bladder scan could also be used to determine whether the bladder is full.

It can take 8 hours for the bladder to regain sensation after epidural analgesia. Women who have had spinal or epidural analgesia for operative delivery should have an indwelling catheter for at least 12 hours

Women with any of the following conditions are at risk of acute urinary retention:

- difficult vaginal birth with perineal/vulval trauma and suturing
- prolonged labour
- epidural analgesia during labour

- vaginal or postoperative abdominal pain
- history of voiding problems

Care of the baby

See Chapter 21.

The placenta

The placenta should be examined and the findings documented. The following checks should be performed:

- ☐ What is the overall appearance: normal/gritty/small or large?
- ☐ Are the cotyledons complete?
- ☐ Are the membranes complete or ragged?
- ☐ Is the insertion of the cord vessels normal or abnormal?

In some cases – such as twin births, stillbirths and other adverse outcomes – it may be advisable to send the placenta for histopathological examination.

Documentation

The midwife is responsible for seeing that all observations are made and recorded before transfer to the postnatal ward:

- case notes (mother and baby)
- birth register
- maternity information system (computer)

Any deviations from normal should be reported to the obstetrician on duty.

21 Care of the newborn

> ! For the majority of infants, the needs after delivery are a warm welcome, clear airways, and vigilance.

No benefits have been demonstrated for the routine suctioning of the newborn's oral and nasal passages. However, if there has been any indication of meconium-stained amniotic fluid then the paediatrician should be called to delivery and the airways cleared under direct vision. The oropharynx should always be cleared before the nasal passages. The aspiration of meconium from the nose and mouth of the unborn baby while the head is still on the perineum is not recommended.

Skin-to-skin contact

The benefits of skin-to-skin contact are:

- maintenance of the baby's body temperature
- more successful breastfeeding

The mother, regardless of whether she intends to breastfeed or formula-feed, should be encouraged to have skin-to-skin contact with the infant immediately following delivery. If the mother is not in a position to do this, the partner may be able to offer skin-to-skin contact.

Skin-to-skin contact may be delayed where there are concerns about the wellbeing of the mother or baby, but it should not be delayed or interrupted by routine procedures such as weighing the baby.

For a baby requiring resuscitation, skin-to-skin contact should be established once the baby has been resuscitated.

The first feed is given once the baby shows signs of readiness (sucking, rooting and hand-to-mouth movements).

Skin-to-skin contact (or its refusal) should be documented.

Prevention of hypothermia

Hypothermia is a core temperature of less than 35°C. Heat loss is more rapid and consequences are more severe in immature babies.

The ideal delivery-suite environment for a baby is:

- still air
- temperature 34°C
- 100% relative humidity

Therefore:

- Optimize the temperature.
- Ensure that the room is not draughty.
- Dry the baby at birth and wrap in a dry towel.
- If resuscitation is required, use a Resuscitaire (i.e. place the baby under radiant heat).

Vitamin K

Vitamin K prophylaxis at birth prevents bleeding due to vitamin K deficiency (formerly known as haemorrhagic disease of the newborn). Information regarding the use of vitamin K should be given to all mothers. Valid parental consent should be obtained and documented.

Routes of administration

- **Intramuscular**: vitamin K 1 mg IM. This is inexpensive and easy to administer. There was some concern about possible links with childhood cancer, but further studies found no link between vitamin K and cancer. Parenteral injection in premature babies is associated with an increased risk of kernicterus, so babies weighing less than 1500 g should receive the lower dose of 0.5 mg IM.
- **Oral**: Konakion MM Paediatric, 2 mg at birth and 2 mg within the next 7 days. For breastfed babies, a further 2 mg dose is given at 1 month; this dose is omitted in formula-fed babies because formula feeds contain vitamin K.

Standard practice is to use the injectable vitamin K preparation. Where parents opt for the oral preparation, refer to patient group direction.

If oral vitamin K has been chosen by a breastfeeding mother then adequate arrangements should be made between the midwife, health visitor, GP and parents to ensure that the third dose is given at 1 month.

Vitamin K is indicated particularly in babies of women who have taken anticonvulsants (e.g. phenytoin) or oral anticoagulants in pregnancy.

Identification of the baby

The delivering/supervising midwife is responsible for ensuring that the baby is wearing an identification band before leaving the labour ward.

An identifying band should be attached securely to each ankle of the baby. This should be done in the presence of the mother if possible. The baby's name and the mother's hospital number should be written clearly on each band.

Breastfeeding

This should be encouraged as soon as possible after delivery.

Management of hypoglycaemia

Hypoglycaemia is a blood glucose level < 2.7 mmol/L.

The following are associated with an increased risk of hypoglycaemia:

- preterm birth
- small for gestational age (below the third centile)
- macrosomia
- diabetic mother
- hypothermia

Signs include cold, sweatiness, jitteriness, behaviour changes, floppiness, apnoea, cyanosis and pallor. Babies with any of these signs should have their blood glucose measured.

Urgent action is required:

☐ Inform the paediatrician.
☐ Give glucose as prescribed by the paediatrician. The baby may have to be transferred to the SCBU.

Preventive care

Babies small for gestational age, and other babies at increased risk, should have:

- feeding (within 2 hours of delivery)
- feeding (3-hourly)
- glucose checked (dipstick) before each feed in the first 48 hours

22 Meconium-stained amniotic fluid

Risk to baby

The baby is at risk of meconium aspiration syndrome. The risk is more significant when there is thick meconium.

Note

Amnioinfusion is not recommended for the management of meconium-stained amniotic fluid.

Meconium-stained fluid in labour

- ☐ Inform the paediatrician.
- ☐ Prepare Resuscitaire and endotracheal tubes.
- ☐ Obtain a CTG.

Meconium-stained fluid at vaginal delivery

Do not suck the mouth and nostrils prior to birth of the shoulders and trunk. You can do so after birth, but only if the baby has thick meconium in the oropharynx. Aspiration of meconium from the nose and mouth of the unborn baby while the head is still on the perineum is not recommended.

If the baby is pink, vigorous and not in respiratory distress then no further resuscitation is necessary.

If the baby is floppy at birth then visualize the vocal cord (by laryngoscopy) and suck if necessary.

If no meconium is seen below the cord and the Apgar score at 5 minutes is greater than 8 and the baby is asymptomatic:

- Observe on the postnatal ward – respiration, feeding and finger-prick glucose.
- The paediatrician should review at 1–2 hours.
- The following observations should be recorded at 1 hour, 2 hours and then 2-hourly for 10 hours:
  - o general wellbeing
  - o chest movements and nasal flare
  - o skin colour, including perfusion by testing capillary refill

- o feeding
- o muscle tone
- o temperature
- o heart rate and respiration.

Admit into SCBU for observation if:

- meconium is seen below the cord
- there is respiratory distress
- the baby is still floppy at 5 minutes

If the mother has had pethidine in the last 4 hours, give naloxone to the baby and observe for 10 minutes. If the baby is still floppy, admit to SCBU.

Check cord blood gases.

Meconium-stained fluid at caesarean section

Transfer immediately to Resuscitaire. The principles are then the same as above.

23 Neonatal resuscitation

All midwives, obstetricians and paediatricians have a responsibility to achieve and maintain the skills needed for neonatal resuscitation.

A list of equipment and drugs is kept in the delivery rooms, obstetric theatre and on Resuscitaires.

All delivery rooms, obstetric theatres and Resuscitaires must be checked daily and before use.

All equipment and drugs used during resuscitation must be replaced as soon as possible.

Heaters should be turned on and warm towels should be readily available.

Principles

At the onset of acute hypoxia, fetal breathing movements become more rapid. As oxygen levels continue to fall, regular breathing movements cease, since the centres responsible for controlling them are unable to function owing to lack of oxygen. The fetus enters a period known as **primary apnoea.** The heart rate falls but the BP is maintained.

If the hypoxia continues and the fetus is not delivered, gasping activity begins. As the gasps fail to aerate the lungs, they fade away. This is because increasing acidosis and hypoxia interfere with the ability of the heart muscle to function effectively. The gasps eventually cease and the fetus enters **secondary** or **terminal apnoea**.

Infants in primary apnoea will quickly recover if the airway is open and oxygenated blood is transported to the heart and lungs. If the infant is in terminal apnoea, he/she will not recover without intervention and may die despite receiving help. It is not possible to distinguish whether an infant who is not breathing at birth is in primary apnoea and about to gasp or has taken his/her last gasp in utero and is now in terminal apnoea.

> **!** All infants born apnoeic must be presumed to be in terminal apnoea.

Avoid thermal stress

Keep the baby dry and warm: all infants must be dried thoroughly and wrapped in clean, warm towels. Cold stress increases metabolic acidosis.

Airway

Ensure that the airway is clear: the correct position for an infant for *all* resuscitation procedures is the neutral position. Both hyperextension and hypoextension of the neck will obstruct the airways. A prominent occiput will tend to flex the neck if the baby is placed dorsal on a flat surface, so it may be necessary to place a support below the baby's shoulders.

Deep suction of the airways should be avoided for at least 5 minutes after birth, except where there has been a history of meconium-stained amniotic fluid.

Evaluation

The following three criteria should be evaluated in order (Figure 23.1):

- breathing
- heart rate
- colour

Breathing

If the airway is clear and effective breathing has not been established then it will be necessary to provide oxygenation by means of assisted breaths. Weak respiratory efforts should be considered the same as no respiratory effort. Provide *five* inflation breaths to clear lung fluid. These are assisted breaths of about 30 cmH$_2$O for about 2–3 seconds. Once inflation breaths have been given, reassess the heart rate and colour. If the heart rate is increasing and the infant is pink, you have successfully inflated the lungs.

Reassess if effective breathing has not been established and/or the infant is not pink:

- Is the infant's airway clear?
- Are there chest movement when you provide ventilatory breaths?
- Has the heart rate picked up?

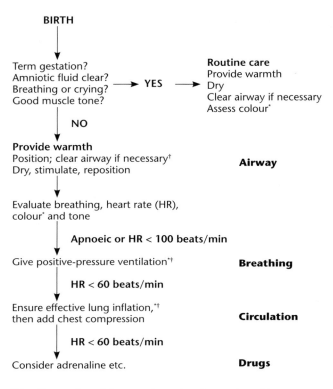

BIRTH

Term gestation?
Amniotic fluid clear? ⟶ **YES** ⟶
Breathing or crying?
Good muscle tone?

Routine care
Provide warmth
Dry
Clear airway if necessary
Assess colour*

NO

Provide warmth
Position; clear airway if necessary†   **Airway**
Dry, stimulate, reposition

Evaluate breathing, heart rate (HR),
colour* and tone

Apnoeic or HR < 100 beats/min

Give positive-pressure ventilation*†   **Breathing**

HR < 60 beats/min

Ensure effective lung inflation,*†
then add chest compression   **Circulation**

HR < 60 beats/min

Consider adrenaline etc.   **Drugs**

*Consider supplemental oxygen at any stage if cyanosis persists
†Tracheal intubation may be considered at several steps

Figure 23.1 Algorithm for neonatal resuscitation. Reproduced with permission from Resuscitation Council (UK). *Resuscitation Guidelines 2005*. London: Resuscitation Council (UK), 2005

If the heart rate does not increase, and the chest does not passively move with each inflation breath, then the airway is probably not clear, so confirm that the baby is in the neutral position and exclude an obstruction in the oropharynx.

If the heart rate remains slow or absent following five inflation breaths, despite good passive chest movement, start chest compression.

Chest compression

In this event, chest compression will be necessary to support circulation until effective oxygenation and pulmonary blood flow are established.

- **Call for help** (paediatric assistance bleep ...).
- Grip the chest in both hands, placing the thumbs together at the front and the fingers over the spine.
- Position the thumbs in the midline just below an imaginary line joining the nipples.
- Compress the chest, aiming to halve the distance between the sternum and the spine.
- Pause briefly between each compression. Aim for 40–60 compressions/min.
- Reassess heart rate every 30 seconds. Continue compression until the pulse rate is 80 beats/min.
- The conventional ratio is three compressions to one inflation breath.
- If there is no response to adequate compression and lung inflation then it may be necessary to administer drugs via an umbilical venous catheter (standard doses of adrenaline given via the tracheal tube are unlikely to be effective). Usually drugs are required only in the most critically distressed infant. See below.
- Midwives may administer only vitamin K and naloxone (patient group directions).
- Check umbilical cord blood gases.

Drugs used in neonatal resuscitation

Adrenaline (1 : 10 000 solution)

Dose: 10 µg/kg (0.1 mL/kg of 1 : 10 000 solution). Additional doses up to 30 µg/kg (0.3 ml/kg of 1 : 10 000 solution) may be given.

Sodium bicarbonate (ideally 4.2% solution)

Dose: 1–2 mmol/kg (2–4 mL/kg of 4.2% solution).

Glucose (10%)

Dose: 250 mg/kg (2.5 mL/kg of 10% glucose).

Note

Resuscitation should take account of the circumstances of the particular neonate. If, for example, there is evidence that the baby has lost blood, isotonic crystalloid may be needed to increase cardiac output.

24 Babies born before arrival at hospital

Babies born before arrival at hospital have relatively high morbidity rates owing to immaturity and low birth weight. The main risk, irrespective of birth weight, is hypothermia.

Some deliveries without medical or midwifery assistance take place at home. These should be managed according to local protocol, and transfer to hospital is not always necessary. Others will happen on the way to hospital or elsewhere outside the home.

There may be background psychosocial problems, which should be addressed where possible. In some cases, the pregnancy has been concealed or there has been no antenatal care.

Mother

☐ Has the placenta been delivered? Is it complete?
☐ Is the uterus firmly retracted?
☐ Is there PPH?
☐ Are there any genital tract lacerations needing repair?
☐ What are BP, pulse and temperature?
☐ Are there any obstetric, medical or social problems?

Baby

☐ Ensure that the baby is warm.
☐ Check colour, breathing and heart rate; call the paediatrician if indicated.
☐ What is the birth weight?
☐ Administer vitamin K, with the mother's consent.

25 Episiotomy

Indications for episiotomy include:

- preventive action when a perineal tear is imminent
- expedition of delivery in cases of fetal distress or maternal exhaustion
- instrumental delivery
- shoulder dystocia (see p. 220)

Episiotomy should not be offered *routinely* at vaginal birth following previous third- or fourth-degree trauma.

Both the indication for episiotomy and the woman's assent should be documented in the labour records. A right mediolateral incision should be used (a midline incision increases the danger of damage to the anal sphincter).

Midwives who have been instructed in perineal repair may undertake the suturing of first- and second-degree tears and episiotomies using 2/0 Vicryl Rapide as suture material. The perineum is infiltrated with 1% lidocaine, the total amount not exceeding 20 mL.

Episiotomies should be repaired as soon as possible after completion of the third stage of labour, preferably by the person who has delivered the baby. Subcuticular suturing is preferable to interrupted suturing of the perineal skin, since it is associated with less pain.

For guidelines on the repair of perineal tears, see Chapter 47.

The following should be documented:

☐ the extent of the tear
☐ the type of suture
☐ vaginal and rectal examination at the end of the procedure
☐ the swabs, sharps and instruments counted at the end of the procedure, and the fact that they are complete

---

Plain fact

In the USA (where a midline episiotomy is cut), the rate of episiotomy with all vaginal deliveries decreased from 60.9% in 1979 to 24.5% in 2004. Anal sphincter laceration with spontaneous vaginal delivery declined from 5% in 1979 to 3.5% in 2004.

26 The woman with a history of childhood sexual abuse

General measures

- Give reassurance.
- Provide the woman with a sense of control.
- Assure her that you will respect her wishes.
- The presence of a support person can be very helpful.

Communication

Choose your words carefully. Some words may bring back sad memories. Maintain confidentiality.

Physical examination and procedures

- Minimize internal examinations.
- Find out if anything can be done to make the examination or procedure less stressful. For example, the woman may wish to take up a particular position or avoid the dorsal position.
- Let the woman know that she can stop the examination or procedure at any time if she finds it too uncomfortable.
- Handle the following with extra sensitivity:
  - o performing an episiotomy
  - o repairing an episiotomy or tear
  - o lithotomy position.

Flashbacks

These may manifest as a panic attack, hyperventilation, a facial expression or a subtle change in body language. Be alert to non-verbal cues.

27 Use of birthing pool

The birthing pool may be used for one or both of the following:

- immersion during the active phase of labour
- delivery of the baby under water

Some women may feel a therapeutic benefit from immersion during labour, but delivery under water carries uncommon but significant risks to the baby, including drowning, respiratory problems, bleeding from a ruptured cord and waterborne infection.

Women using the birthing pool should be looked after only by midwives who have acquired the requisite skills and confidence.

Inclusion criteria

☐   37 completed weeks
☐   normal pregnancy
☐   singleton fetus with cephalic presentation
☐   no systemic sedation
☐   spontaneous rupture of membranes <24 hours
☐   normal observations: pulse, temperature and BP
☐   normal CTG

Exclusion criteria

- APH
- induction of labour
- meconium-stained amniotic fluid
- IUGR
- multiple pregnancy
- malpresentation
- previous CS
- medical conditions: diabetes, epilepsy, HIV, group B streptococcus, etc.
- any condition requiring continuous fetal monitoring
- mother requiring IV cannula
- macrosomic baby
- opioid analgesia taken in the last 2 hours

Conduct of labour

The pool

- The water depth should be such that the woman's torso is exposed (i.e. not immersed), to facilitate thermoregulation through evaporation.
- The water should be free of debris during delivery.
- The floor of the pool room should be dry.
- The temperature should not exceed 37.5°C. Check the temperature of the pool and the woman hourly, and aim for a pool temperature of 32–36°C during labour and 36–37°C at delivery. If the woman's temperature increases by 1°C above the baseline recording, she should be advised to leave the pool.

Analgesia

Entonox may be used. If pethidine or an epidural is required, the mother will have to leave the pool.

Progress of labour

- Monitor the fetal heart rate using underwater Doppler ultrasound.
- Vaginal examinations should be performed out of the pool.
- Progress should be recorded on the partogram.

Support in labour

- The woman should not be left on her own at any time.
- Give liberal oral fluids and avoid dehydration.

Delivery

- Two midwives should be present at delivery.
- If the woman raises herself out of the water and exposes the fetal head to air, once the presenting part is visible, she should be advised to remain out of the water to avoid the risk of premature gasping under water.
- Do not perform an episiotomy or cut the cord under water.
- If the baby is delivered in water, ensure that the head is the first part to emerge from the water.
- The third stage, whether active or physiological, must be performed out of water.

General

The usual infection control, handling and moving, and health and safety standards apply. Local protocols should be agreed with the microbiology and relevant governance teams. This includes guidance on the prevention of *Legionella* build-up in the water supply, particularly in seldomly used pools.

Further reading for Part II

Prelabour rupture of membranes at term (37–42 weeks)

Bricker L, Peden H, Tomlinson AJ et al. Titrated low-dose vaginal and/or oral misoprostol to induce labour for prelabour membrane rupture: a randomised trial. *BJOG* 2008; **115**: 1503–11.

Calder AA, Loughney AD, Weir CJ, Barber JW. Induction of labour in nulliparous and multiparous women: a UK, multicentre, open-label study of intravaginal misoprostol in comparison with dinoprostone. *BJOG* 2008; **115**: 1279–88.

Dare MR, Middleton P, Crowther CA et al. Planned early birth versus expectant management (waiting) for prelabour rupture of membranes at term (37 weeks or more). *Cochrane Database Syst Rev* 2006; (1): CD005302.

Flenady V, King JF. Antibiotics for prelabour rupture of membranes at or near term. *Cochrane Database Syst Rev* 2002; (3): CD001807.

Morris JM, Roberts CL, Crowther CA, Buchanan SL, Henderson-Smart DJ, Salkeld G. Protocol for the immediate delivery versus expectant care of women with preterm prelabour rupture of the membranes close to term (PPROMT) Trial [ISRCTN44485060]. *BMC Pregnancy Childbirth* 2006; **6**: 9.

Management of the first stage of labour

Albers LL, Anderson D, Cragin L et al. The relationship of ambulation in labor to operative delivery. *J Nurse Midwifery* 1997; **42**: 4–8.

American College of Nurse–Midwives. Providing oral nutrition to women in labor. *J Midwifery Womens Health* 2008; **53**: 276–83.

Andrews CM, Chrzanowski M. Maternal position, labour and comfort. *Appl Nurs Res* 1990; **3**: 7–13.

Caldeyro-Barcia R, Noriega-Guerra L, Cibils LA et al. Effect of position changes on the intensity and frequency of uterine contractions during labor. *Am J Obstet Gynecol* 1960; **80**: 284–90.

Hodnett ED, Gates S, Hofmeyr GJ, Sakala C. Continuous support for women during childbirth. *Cochrane Database Syst Rev* 2007; (3): CD003766.

Newton C, Beere P. Oral intake in labour: Nottingham's policy formulated and audited. *Br J Midwifery* 1997; **5**: 418–22.

National Institute for Health and Clinical Excellence (NICE). *Intrapartum Care: Care of Healthy Women and their Babies during Childbirth.* NICE Clinical Guideline 55. London: NICE, September 2007. Available at: www.nice.org.uk/nicemedia/pdf/IPCNICEGuidance.pdf.

O'Sullivan G, Liu B, Shennan AH. Oral intake during labor. *Int Anesthesiol Clin* 2007; **45**: 133–47.

Fetal monitoring

Gibb D, Arulkumaran S. *Fetal Monitoring in Practice,* 3rd edn. Edinburgh: Churchill Livingstone, 2008.

K2 Medical Systems. *Fetal Monitoring Training System* (software). Plymouth: K2 Medical Systems. Available at: www.k2ms.com.

McIntosh MCM. Continuous fetal heart rate monitoring: Is there a conflict between confidential enquiry findings and results of randomised trials? *J R Soc Med* 2001; **94**: 14–16.

National Institute for Health and Clinical Excellence (NICE). *Intrapartum Care: Care of Healthy Women and their Babies during Childbirth.* NICE Clinical Guideline 55. London: NICE, September 2007. Available at: www.nice.org.uk/nicemedia/pdf/ IPCNICEGuidance.pdf.

Fetal scalp blood sampling

Gibb D. Intrapartum care. In: Clements RV, ed. *Risk Management and Litigation in Obstetrics and Gynaecology.* London: RSM Press, 2001: 167–203.

Wiberg-Itzel E, Lipponer C, Norman M et al. Determination of pH or lactate in fetal scalp blood in management of intrapartum fetal distress: randomised controlled multicentre trial. *BMJ* 2008; **336**: 1284–7.

Augmentation of labour

Cheek TG, Samuels P, Miller F et al. Normal saline i.v. fluid decreases uterine activity in active labour. *Br J Anaesth* 1996; **77**: 632–5.

Smyth RMD, Alldred SK, Markham C. Amniotomy for shortening spontaneous labour. *Cochrane Database Syst Rev* 2007; (4): CD006167.

Patka JH, Lodolce AE, Johnston AK. High- versus low-dose oxytocin for augmentation or induction of labor. *Ann Pharmacother* 2005; **39**: 95–101.

Epidural analgesia in labour

Association of Anaesthetists of Great Britain and Ireland and Obstetric Anaesthetists' Association. *OAA/AAGBI Guidelines for Obstetric Anaesthesia Services,* Revised Edition 2005. London: AAGBI and OAA, May 2005. Available at: www.aagbi.org/publications/guidelines/docs/obstetric05.pdf.

Campbell DC, Tran T. Conversion of epidural labour analgesia to epidural anesthesia for intrapartum cesarean delivery. *Can J Anaesth* 2009; **56**: 19–26.

Horlocker TT, Heit JA. Low molecular weight heparin: biochemistry, pharmacology, peri-operative prophylaxis regimens, and guidelines for regional anaesthetic management. *Anesth Analg* 1997; **85**: 874–85.

Litwin AA. Mode of delivery following labor epidural analgesia: influence of ropivacaine and bupivacaine. *Am Assoc Nurse Anesth J* 2001; **69**: 259–61.

Torvaldsen S, Roberts CL, Bell JC, Raynes-Greenow CH. Discontinuation of epidural analgesia late in labour for reducing the adverse delivery outcomes associated with epidural analgesia. *Cochrane Database Syst Rev* 2004; (4): CD004457.

Management of the second stage of labour

Altman M, Lydon-Rochelle M. Prolonged second stage of labor and the risk of adverse maternal and perinatal outcomes: a systematic review. *Birth* 2006; **33**: 315–22.

Brancato RM, Church S, Stone PW. A meta-analysis of passive descent versus immediate pushing in nulliparous women with epidural analgesia in the second stage of labor. *J Obstet Gynecol Neonatal Nurs* 2008; **37**: 4–12.

Cheng Y, Hopkins L, Caughey A. How long is too long: Does a prolonged second stage of labor in nulliparous women affect maternal and neonatal outcomes? *Am J Obstet Gynecol* 2004; **191**: 933–8.

Stewart KS. The second stage. In: Studd J, ed. *Progress in Obstetrics and Gynaecology*, Vol 4. Edinburgh: Churchill Livingstone, 1984: 197–216.

National Institute for Health and Clinical Excellence (NICE). *Intrapartum Care: Care of Healthy Women and their Babies during Childbirth*. NICE Clinical Guideline 55. London: NICE, September 2007. Available at: www.nice.org.uk/nicemedia/pdf/IPCNICEGuidance.pdf.

Management of the third stage of labour

McDonald S. Physiology and management of the third stage of labour. In: Fraser D, Cooper M, eds. *Myles' Textbook for Midwives*, 15th edn. London: Churchill Livingstone, 2009: Chap 29.

Prendiville WJP, Elbourne D, McDonald SJ. Active versus expectant management in the third stage of labour. *Cochrane Database Syst Rev* 2000; (3): CD000007.

Rogers J, Wood J, McCandish R et al. Active versus expectant management of the third stage of labour: the Hinchingbrooke randomised controlled trial. *Lancet* 1998; **351**: 693–9.

Immediate postpartum care

Christensson K, Siles C, Moreno L et al. Temperature, metabolic adaptation and crying in healthy full-term newborns cared for skin-to-skin or in a cot. *Acta Paediatr* 1992; **81**: 488–93.

Moore ER, Anderson GC, Bergman N. Early skin-to-skin contact for mothers and their healthy newborn infants. *Cochrane Database Syst Rev* 2007; (3): CD003519.

Care of the newborn

Dear P, Newell S. *Neonatology for the MRCOG*. London: RCOG Press, 1996.

Royal College of Midwives. *Vitamin K*. Position Paper 13b. London: Royal College of Midwives, 1999. Available at: www.library.nhs.uk/GUIDELINESFINDER/ViewResource.aspx?resID=29756.

Van Winckel M, De Bruyne R, Van De Velde S, Van Biervliet S. Vitamin K, an update for the paediatrician. *Eur J Pediatr* 2009; **168**: 127–34.

Meconium-stained amniotic fluid

Vain NE, Szyld EG, Prudent LM et al. Oropharyngeal and nasopharyngeal suctioning of meconium-stained neonates before delivery of their shoulders: multicentre, randomised controlled trial. *Lancet* 2004; **364**: 597–602.

Wiswell TE, Gannon CM, Jacob J et al. Delivery room management of the apparently vigorous meconium-stained neonate: results of the multicenter international collaborative trial. *Pediatrics* 2000; **105**: 1–7.

Xu H, Mas-Calvet M, Wei SQ, Luo ZC, Fraser WD. Abnormal fetal heart rate tracing patterns in patients with thick meconium staining of the amniotic fluid: association with perinatal outcomes. *Am J Obstet Gynecol* 2009; **200**: 283.e1–7.

Neonatal resuscitation

Morley CJ, Davis PG. Advances in neonatal resuscitation: supporting transition. *Arch Dis Child Fetal Neonatal Ed* 2008; **93**: F334–6.

Richmond S. Newborn life support. In: *Resuscitation Guidelines 2005*. Resuscitation Council (UK), December 2005: 97–104. Available at www.resus.org.uk/pages/nls.pdf.

Babies born before arrival at hospital

Bhoopalam PS, Watkinson M. Babies born before arrival at hospital. *Br J Obstet Gynaecol* 1991; **98**: 57–64.

Rodie VA, Thomson AJ, Norman JE. Accidental out-of-hospital deliveries: an obstetric and neonatal case control study. *Acta Obstet Gynecol Scand*. 2002; **81**: 50-4.

Repair of episiotomy and first-/second-degree perineal repair

Kettle C, Hills RK, Ismail KMK. Continuous versus interrupted sutures for repair of episiotomy or second degree tears. *Cochrane Database Syst Rev* 2007; (4): CD000947.

The woman with a history of childhood sexual abuse

Rhodes N, Hutchinson S. Labor experiences of childhood sexual abuse survivors. *Birth* 1994; **21**: 213–20.

Tidy H. Care for survivors of childhood sexual abuse. *Mod Midwife* 1996; **6**: 17–19.

Leeners B, Neumaier-Wagner P, Quarg AF, Rath W. Childhood sexual abuse (CSA) experiences: an underestimated factor in perinatal care. *Acta Obstet Gynecol Scand* 2006; **85**: 971–6.

Leeners B, Richter-Appelt H, Imthurn B, Rath W. Influence of childhood sexual abuse on pregnancy, delivery, and the early postpartum period in adult women. *J Psychosom Res* 2006; **61**: 139–51.

Use of birthing pool

Cluett ER, Nikodem VC, McCandlish RE, Burns EE. Immersion in water in pregnancy, labour and birth. *Cochrane Database Syst Rev* 2004; (2): CD000111.

Steer PJ, Deans AC. Labour and birth in water: temperature of pool is important. *BMJ* 1995; **311**: 390–1.

Royal College of Obstetricians and Gynaecologists/Royal College of Midwives. *Joint Statement No.1: Immersion in Water during Labour and Birth.* Issued April 2006. Available at: www.rcog.org.uk/files/rcog-corp/uploaded-files/JointStatmentBirthInWater2006.pdf.

PART III
Abnormal and high-risk labour

Formal risk assessment and contingency planning should start antenatally – but should not end there. Each clinical episode offers an opportunity to reassess and contain risk.

28 Caesarean section

Preparations

- ☐ Obtain consent. A competent pregnant woman is entitled to decline CS, even if her life or that of the baby is at risk.
- ☐ Group-and-save or cross-match, as required. Blood should be cross-matched if any of the following apply:
  - maternal anaemia ([Hb] < 10 g/dL)
  - placenta praevia (cross-match 4 units)
  - anterior placenta and previous CS
  - any other situation where higher than usual blood loss is anticipated (e.g. a clotting disorder or large fibroids).
- ☐ Insert a cannula (size 16G).
- ☐ Perform a risk assessment for DVT prophylaxis (see the protocol on p. 169).
- ☐ It is mandatory for the woman to fast for at least 6 hours before an elective CS. She may drink water (150 mL) up to 2 hours before elective surgery.
- ☐ In the case of CS for breech presentation (elective or emergency), always confirm by means of an ultrasound scan that the presentation is still breech.

In theatre:

- ☐ Catheterize the bladder (if not already done).
- ☐ Check fetal heart tones.
- ☐ Place the patient in the left lateral tilt (15°).

Medication to reduce the risk of aspiration syndrome

- ☐ Ranitidine 150 mg orally on the night of admission and at 0730 the following day. For emergencies, check whether ranitidine was given in labour (oral ranitidine 150 mg is effective if given at least 60 minutes before CS). If not, give ranitidine 50 mg in 20 mL 0.9% saline IV, over 2 minutes.
- ☐ Metoclopramide 10 mg orally.
- ☐ Sodium citrate 30 mL orally.

Classification of urgency of CS

- **Emergency – to be performed immediately**:
  - immediate threat to life of woman or fetus
  - massive APH
  - cord prolapse
  - placental abruption
  - profound unresponsive fetal bradycardia
  - fetal distress (pH ≤ 7.20)
  - uterine rupture.
- **Urgent**: maternal or fetal compromise that is not immediately life-threatening (e.g. failure to progress).
- **Scheduled**: needing early delivery but no immediate maternal or fetal compromise (e.g. IUGR with abnormal Doppler).
- **Elective**: at a time to suit the woman and the maternity team, e.g. previous CS.

When CS becomes a probability for a woman in labour, she should be informed and the anaesthetist should be alerted. This may allow discussion with the woman in less pressing circumstances.

Elective CS

- To reduce the risk of respiratory distress in the newborn, elective CS should not be performed routinely before 39 weeks' gestation. In selected cases, it will be sensible to schedule the operation earlier than this. For example, it may be safer to have a planned CS at 38 weeks for a woman with placenta praevia or three previous CS than have this woman present in labour a few days before a CS booked for 39 weeks.
- Book with the labour ward as directed by local protocol.
- There should be a maximum of three cases per session (two cases, if complicated).
- If the woman falls into any of the following categories, the list should be covered by the consultant anaesthetist:
  - previous anaesthetic complications
  - obesity (body mass index > 30 kg/m² at booking)
  - multiple pregnancy
  - placenta praevia
  - hypertensive disease
  - diabetes mellitus
  - Jehovah's Witness
  - significant coexisting disease (cardiac, renal or respiratory).

- Low-risk patients can be admitted on the day of operation, but bloods and consent must be obtained in clinic, ranitidine prescribed, and the patient told to starve from midnight.

Emergency CS

☐ Contact the consultant on duty/call (in their absence, contact any other consultant).

☐ Obtain consent.

☐ Classify and document the urgency of the operation (see the classification above).

☐ Notify:
- the operating department practitioner (ODP)
- the anaesthetist (specify the urgency of the operation)
- the paediatrician.

☐ FBC, group-and-save or cross-match as required.

☐ Discontinue Syntocinon (oxytocin) infusion, if in progress.

☐ Ensure that thromboprophylaxis is administered.

Surgical procedure

☐ The procedure is performed with the patient in a left lateral tilt.

☐ Bleeps should not be brought into the theatre. If a bleep goes off in theatre during induction of general anaesthesia or while the patient is under regional analgesia, it could be alarming to the patient and/or her partner. There could also be breach of confidentiality when messages are passed to the doctor.

☐ The woman should be accorded due respect and dignity throughout the operation. This means, for example, that she is unclothed only as and when necessary, noise and frivolous side conversations are minimized, and the operation field is screened from view. Her partner should also be supported.

☐ The uterus should not be exteriorized as routine.

☐ Spontaneous separation of the placenta followed by cord traction is preferable to manual removal of the placenta. Manual removal is associated with increased blood loss and postpartum endometritis.

☐ Cord blood gas analysis should be performed following CS for fetal distress.

☐ Prophylactic antibiotics should be given after clamping the cord (see below).

Prophylactic antibiotics

Antibiotics given prophylactically reduce the incidence of postpartum endometritis.

The antibiotic is administered after the umbilical cord has been clamped: cefuroxime IV 750 mg and metronidazole IV 500 mg immediately.

If the woman is allergic to penicillin then give erythromycin 1 g.

High-risk cases

A consultant or suitably experienced senior doctor should be present for CS performed for the following indications/circumstances:

- placenta praevia
- placental abruption
- multiple previous CS
- body mass index > 35 kg/m^2
- delivery < 32 weeks
- any other potentially complicated CS

Delayed elective CS

- Keep the woman and her partner informed of events.
- If the operation is delayed by more than 4 hours, start an IV infusion.

Postoperative care

Give analgesia as required.

The woman should be monitored by an appropriately trained member of staff until she is stable and able to communicate. See Chapter 29. Respiratory rate, heart rate, BP, pain and sedation should be recorded every half-hour for 4 hours, then 4-hourly. The use of an EWS (see p. 87) is recommended.

If CS was done under regional block, the indwelling bladder catheter should remain in place until the woman is ambulant, to prevent bladder over-distension.

Ensure that thromboprophylaxis has been prescribed/ administered. LMWH can be commenced 6 hours after spinal anaesthesia, and 8 hours after epidural analgesia (see p. 172 and 179).

29 Recovery of obstetric patients

All patients should be recovered in a designated fully staffed and equipped recovery area. They should be under continuous clinical observation for at least 30 minutes:

- ☐ continuous ECG
- ☐ pulse oximetry
- ☐ BP monitoring

The following should be documented:

- ☐ level of consciousness
- ☐ pulse rate
- ☐ temperature
- ☐ pain score
- ☐ BP
- ☐ O_2 saturation
- ☐ respiratory rate
- ☐ blood loss from wound (and from drain, if present)
- ☐ IV infusions
- ☐ blood loss from vagina
- ☐ drugs administered

The frequency of observations will depend on the stage of recovery and the clinical condition of the patient, but vital signs should be recorded at least every 15 minutes in the first hour.

Discharge from the recovery area should be according to a protocol agreed by the anaesthetist.

Before transfer to the postnatal ward, all patients must:

- be easily rousable
- have full airway control
- have adequate pain relief
- have normal observations
- have IV fluids, antiemetics and analgesia prescribed as required

---

! Midwifery staff deputed to look after postoperative patients should be specifically trained in monitoring, care of the airway and resuscitative procedures and should be supervised by a defined anaesthetist at all times.

UK Health Departments. *Report on Confidential Enquiries into Maternal Deaths in the United Kingdom 1988–1990*. London: HMSO, 1994

30 High-dependency care

High-dependency care is indicated in the following circumstances:

- when there is haemodynamic instability (due to hypovolaemia, haemorrhage or sepsis)
- when a continuous ECG is required
- for invasive pressure monitoring (central venous pressure or arterial line)
- when there is acute impairment of respiratory, renal or metabolic function

One or more of the above is likely to happen in cases of:

- major PPH
- fulminating pre-eclampsia
- eclampsia
- DIC
- pulmonary oedema
- cardiac failure
- cardiomyopathy
- sudden maternal collapse
- septicaemia

All observations and results of investigations must be recorded in a high-dependency chart.

Some patients may need to be transferred to the general HDU or ICU of the hospital. This should be done in consultation with both the consultant anaesthetist and the consultant obstetrician (see also p. 13). Timely transfer to ICU is associated with a better outcome; conversely, delayed transfer has contributed to maternal death in some cases reviewed by the Confidential Enquiries into Maternal Deaths in the United Kingdom.

Early Warning Score

The Confidential Enquiries into Maternal Deaths in the UK recommended the use of obstetric early warning charts for monitoring high-risk cases.

An example of an EWS grid is provided in Table 30.1. The selection of cases, frequency of recording and who to call for various levels of EWS should be according to local protocols.

Table 30.1 A matrix for determining Early Warning Score.

Score	3	2	1	0	1	2	3
Temp	–	≤35.0	35.1–36.0	36.1–37.9	38.0–38.9	≥39.0	–
Systolic BP	≤70	71–80	81–100	101–139	–	140–159	≥160
Diastolic BP	–	–	–	<90	90–109	–	≥110
HR	–	≤40	41–50	51–100	101–110	111–129	≥130
RR	–	≤8	–	9–14	15–20	21–29	≥30
CNS	–	–	–	Alert	Voice	Pain	Unresponsive
%SaO$_2$	–	–	–	–	–	–	≤92 air or ≤95 in O$_2$

EWS = 6: High risk of deterioration

EWS = 4–5: Medium risk of deterioration

EWS = 3: Low risk of deterioration

Scores between 3 and 6 should trigger action as directed in the local protocol. For an example of a colour graph used to record EWS. Adapted from Swanton RDJ, Al-Rawi S, Weea MYK. A national survey of obstetric early warning systems in the United Kingdom. *International Journal of Obstetric Anesthesia* 2009;**18**:253–257. doi:10.1016/j.ijoa.2009.01.008

31 Failed intubation drill

The incidence of failed intubation is higher in obstetric anaesthesia than in the general population. In one UK region, the incidence was 1 in 238 anaesthetics and in half of the cases reviewed there was a failure to follow an accepted protocol for failed tracheal intubation.

There should be no more than two attempts at intubation. Repeated attempts increase the chances of aspiration. For the second attempt, use a bougie or smaller tracheal tubes and/or McCoy laryngoscope as appropriate. Failed intubation causes no harm to the mother as long as oxygenation is maintained.

☐ Call for help.
☐ Maintain cricoid pressure.
☐ Keep the patient in a supine position with left lateral tilt.
☐ Give oxygen via a facemask.
☐ If successful, await return of spontaneous ventilation, turn the patient and allow her to waken.
☐ If mask ventilation is not possible, attempt insertion of a laryngeal mask airway. (This may require partial release of cricoid pressure.) If successful, turn the patient and allow her to waken.
☐ If laryngeal mask airway insertion is unsuccessful and spontaneous breathing does not return, perform needle cricothyrotomy to maintain oxygenation.

Surgery should proceed only if the mother's life depends on it (e.g. in cardiac arrest or massive haemorrhage). In this case, a spontaneous breathing technique via a facemask or laryngeal mask should be used and cricoid pressure maintained. Sevoflurane is the inhalational agent of choice in this situation.

After waking the patient, the options are regional anaesthesia, local infiltration and awake fibreoptic intubation.

32 Instrumental delivery

Approximately 1 in 10 deliveries in the industrialized world is an instrumental vaginal delivery.

Instrumental delivery carries significant risks of acute and long-term physical and psychological complications for mother and baby. Care should be taken in selecting cases. The need for instrumental delivery could be reduced by provision of one-to-one support in labour, upright or lateral position, use of oxytocin for prolonged second stage in primigravid women, and delayed pushing in women using epidural analgesia.

Avoiding harm

Harm can be avoided if a number of precautions are taken:

- following the advice given above to reduce the rate of instrumental delivery
- careful case selection – knowing when and when not to perform forceps or vacuum-assisted (ventouse) delivery
- use of the right technique
- appropriate management of malrotation
- appropriate management of trial of instrumental delivery
- mindfulness – beware of fixation with achieving vaginal delivery

Indications for instrumental delivery

- fetal distress
- maternal distress or exhaustion
- delayed second stage of labour (see Chapter 17)
- after-coming head at breech delivery
- elective procedure where maternal down-bearing effort is inadvisable:
  - o dural tap at epidural
  - o maternal heart disease
  - o severe pre-eclampsia
  - o respiratory distress
  - o detached retina

Conditions to be fulfilled before instrumental delivery

☐ There is full cervical dilatation.
☐ The bladder has been catheterized.
☐ Presentation is cephalic.
☐ The bony presenting part is at or below the level of the ischial spines.
☐ No more than one-fifth of the fetal head is palpable abdominally.
☐ The position of the presenting part is defined clearly.
☐ The fetal membranes have ruptured.
☐ There is adequate analgesia.
☐ There are good uterine contractions.

It follows from the above that cephalopelvic disproportion, unengaged fetal head and malpresentation (e.g. brow or breech presentation) are contraindications to instrumental delivery. For further contraindications specific to vacuum-assisted delivery, see below.

Classification of instrumental vaginal delivery

The classification of instrumental vaginal delivery according to the American College of Obstetricians and Gynecologists (ACOG) is shown in Table 32.1.

Table 32.1 ACOG classification of instrumental vaginal delivery

Type	Indices
Outlet	• Fetal scalp is visible without separating the labia • Fetal skull has reached the pelvic floor • Sagittal suture is in the anteroposterior diameter or right or left occiput anterior or posterior position (rotation ≤ 45°) • Fetal head is at or on the perineum
Low	• Leading point of the skull (not caput) is at station plus ≥2 cm and not on the pelvic floor • Two subdivisions: (a) rotation ≤ 45° (b) rotation > 45°
Mid	• Fetal head is one-fifth palpable per abdomen • Leading point of the skull is above station plus 2 cm but not above the ischial spines • Two subdivisions: (a) rotation ≤ 45° (b) rotation > 45°
High	Not included in classification

Reproduced with permission from *Operative Vaginal Delivery, Technical Bulletin 196*. Washington, DC: American College of Obstetricians and Gynecologists.

Communication

The woman (and her partner, if present) should be kept informed before and during the procedure:

☐   Warn that an episiotomy may be performed.
☐   For vacuum-assisted delivery, warn to expect a temporary swelling on the baby's head where the cup is applied.

All women having an instrumental delivery should have a left lateral tilt to prevent supine hypotension syndrome.

Choice of instrument

The operator should use an instrument that they are comfortable with.

Forceps should be used where vacuum-assisted delivery is contraindicated (see below). Forceps are also preferable if there is poor or no maternal effort (poor uterine action or the woman is too tired to push).

Vacuum-assisted delivery

Choose the appropriate cup:

• Soft (silicone or plastic) cups should only be used for outlet deliveries and occipito-anterior position with ≤45° rotation.
• For other cases, use a rigid (plastic or metal) cup. For occipito-posterior and occipitotransverse positions, a rigid cup designed for posterior application should be used.

Whichever cup is used, the most important factor in accomplishing safe delivery is correct placement of the cup.

Procedure

A: Ask for help, address the woman, palpate the abdomen and ensure that anaesthesia is adequate.
B: Bladder is empty.
C: Cervix is completely dilated.
D: Determine position.
E: Equipment is ready.
F: 'Flexing median' application of cup. The flexion point, located on the sagittal suture 3 cm in front of the posterior fontanelle,

is a key landmark in vacuum-assisted delivery because if the cup is not applied over this point, deflection of the head and cup detachment are more likely to occur. Sudden detachment may cause scalp injury. The sagittal suture should be centred under the vacuum. Check the vacuum cup to ensure that it does not include maternal tissue.

G: Gentle, steady traction, should be applied at right angles to the cup, the axis of traction following the pelvic curve.

H: Halt the procedure if :
- there has been no descent with three consecutive pulls
- the cup detaches two times, and the head is not on the perineum – cup detachment is associated with rapid compression/decompression forces and should be avoided
- 15 minutes have elapsed since application of the cup (some protocols allow up to 20 minutes).

I: Evaluate for incision. Routine episiotomy is not necessary.

J: Remove the cup when the jaw is visible.

In the following cases, vacuum-assisted delivery may be performed by an experienced obstetrician when the cervix is 9 cm dilated:

- delivery of the second twin
- cord prolapse
- fetal distress with the presenting part below the level of the ischial spines

Contraindications to vacuum-assisted delivery

- fetal thrombocytopenia or clotting disorder
- maternal idiopathic thrombocytopenic purpura
- early preterm labour (<34 weeks) – vacuum should not be used, because of the risk of intracranial haemorrhage, cephalhaematoma and neonatal jaundice, but forceps may be applied
- malpresentation (face or brow)
- cephalopelvic disproportion
- repeated scalp FBS
- fetal head not engaged

Forceps delivery

A–E: as above.

F: The forceps blades are applied and checked. The posterior fontanelle should be located midway between the sides of the blades, with the lambdoid sutures equidistant from the blades and one finger-breadth above the plane of the shanks. A distance greater than this indicates that the head is extended; if the distance is less than one finger-breadth, this indicates that the head is over-flexed. The sagittal suture must be perpendicular to the plane of the shanks throughout its length; the fenestration of the blades should be barely felt, and the amount of fenestration felt on each side should be equal. If the blades have not been applied deeply enough, the palpable fenestration will be more than a fingertip and the operator is alerted to the risk of facial nerve injury.

G: Gentle traction should be applied, as described above. Ease the grip between contractions, to reduce compression of the baby's head.

H: Halt – abandon the procedure if there is no descent with three contractions or pulls or if 15 minutes have elapsed.

! **Caution**

- Do not perform instrumental delivery unless absolutely certain of presentation, the position of the fetal head and cervical dilatation.

- Maternal deaths have been reported from cervical tear when a ventouse cup has been applied before full cervical dilatation.

- In a case where the child sustained brain damage at birth following a ventouse delivery, the High Court ruled that it was negligent for a senior registrar to carry out a vacuum-assisted delivery before the cervix was fully dilated; see Fotedar v St George's Healthcare NHS Trust [2005] EWHC 1327 (QB).

- The operator must be willing to abandon the procedure if there is no descent of the fetal head.

Trial of instrumental delivery

When there are features suggesting that vaginal delivery is feasible but could be difficult, a trial of instrumental delivery is acceptable practice, provided that this is performed in theatre with ready recourse to CS if needed. The features include prolonged labour, one-fifth of the baby's head palpable abdominally, occipitoposterior position, presenting part at the level of the spines, excessive caput, macrosomia and body mass index > 30. Selection of cases is important, and a trial of instrumental delivery is inappropriate where there is obstructed labour. A trial in theatre is not a justification for attempting high forceps delivery.

- ☐ Inform the consultant before proceeding.
- ☐ Inform the anaesthetist and paediatrician.
- ☐ Fully explain the plan to the woman and her partner. Obtain consent for CS to be performed if the trial of instrumental delivery fails. Also, keep the couple informed during the procedure.
- ☐ There should be CTG monitoring while setting up for anaesthesia/delivery, as well as during the interval between an unsuccessful trial and CS.
- ☐ Cord blood analysis (pH and base excess) should be performed.

Decision-making

A trial of instrumental delivery is, as its name suggests, a trial, and proceeding to a CS should not be seen as a failure. There is no room for heroism. If rotation, descent and delivery are not readily accomplished, proceed to CS.

The principle of abandonment

This applies to presumed straightforward instrumental deliveries and those conducted as a trial in theatre.

An attempt at instrumental vaginal delivery should be halted if:

- there is difficulty in applying the instrument
- there is no descent with each pull
- delivery is not imminent following three pulls of a correctly applied instrument
- 15 minutes (or 20 minutes, depending on the local protocol) has elapsed and the baby has not been delivered

If any of the above apply:

- the accoucheur should resist the temptation to try one more time
- a second instrument should not be used

Post-delivery

☐ Ensure that instruments and swabs are accounted for, and document this.

☐ Administer thromboembolism prophylaxis as appropriate.

☐ Give analgesia as appropriate.

☐ Perform a cord blood analysis (pH and base excess).

☐ Examine the baby for any scalp, facial or other injuries.

☐ Recommend vitamin K.

☐ Provide full documentation (see below).

☐ If there are any complications, discuss these with the woman.

☐ Bladder care: observe for urinary retention.

Documentation

The following should be documented:

☐ indication

☐ anaesthesia

☐ instrument(s) used

☐ findings on examination: fifths palpable; position and station of the fetal head, degree of moulding and caput; adequacy of pelvis

☐ procedure, including ease of application of instrument, number of pulls, and number of detachments if any

☐ time of commencement and completion

☐ condition of the baby, including findings on examination

☐ assessment of the vagina and perineum after delivery

☐ findings on rectal examination after delivery

☐ any complications and how they were managed

☐ swab count

☐ cord pH

☐ details of perineal repair, if applicable

The use of a proforma incorporating the above has been shown to improve documentation.

Errors in instrumental vaginal delivery

Table 32.2 shows examples of errors in instrumental vaginal delivery.

Table 32.2 Examples of errors in instrumental vaginal delivery.

Type of error	Description	Possible consequence	Safe practice
A: Action			
Operation omitted	Abdominal palpation not done	Level of presenting part misjudged	Use of proforma/checklist
Operation mistimed	Rotation done during a contraction	Cervical spine injury to the fetus	Rotate only when uterus is relaxed
Operation too long or too short	Prolonged traction	Intracranial injury	Stick to time limits and number of pulls
Operation in wrong direction	Traction directed forwards and upwards too soon; this causes premature extension of the head as a result of which a larger circumference of the head emerges at the introitus	Third degree perineal tear	Mind axis of traction
Operation too much	Continuous traction applied	Compression of fetal head	Only apply traction during a contraction
B: Information retrieval			
Information not retrieved	No assessment regarding thromboprophylaxis	Prophylaxis not prescribed	Incorporate this assessment into documentation proforma
	History of diabetes disregarded	Shoulder dystocia not anticipated	Identify background risk factors before offering instrumental delivery
Wrong information retrieved	Mistaken head level or position Thinking the cervix is fully dilated when it is not	Misapplication of instrument; trauma Cervical tear	Double check
Incomplete information retrieved	Failure to assess moulding Omission of equipment check	Traumatic delivery; brain injury Delay in delivery; stress and impairment of cognition	Adopt systematic approach to assessment
C: Procedural checks			
Check omitted or not properly done	Failure to ensure cup does not catch tissue	Vaginal laceration	Training Understand reason for check
	Check for proper application of forceps not done as described in text	Trauma to baby's face and eye	
	No check for descent with pull	Undue traction applied	Beware of confirmation bias
	PR not done at end of procedure	Third degree tear missed	Include VE, PR, swab check in documentation
	VE not done at end of procedure Swabs not counted	Retained swab in vagina	
D: Communication			
Failure to communicate	With woman	Valid consent not obtained	Verbal and eye contact: empathy
	With midwife	Patient given conflicting information	Preoperative briefing
	With senior colleague	Required supervision not provided	
	With anaesthetist	Inadequate analgesia	Team work
	With paediatrician	Neonatal resuscitation delayed	
E: Selection (choosing from a number of options)			
	Wrong ventouse cup type	Avoidable failure of ventouse	See text
	Ill-advised sequential instrumentation	Neonatal handicap	
F: Cognition			
Failure to anticipate	Failure to anticipate PPH in prolonged labour	Massive haemorrhage	Have Syntocinon infusion ready at delivery
Failure to ask the right questions	No descent despite traction: is position correctly determined? Is pulling in the right direction?	Trauma	Situational awareness
	Forceps have less than secure grip of head: is there undiagnosed OP? Is forceps applied over baby's face?	Trauma	Situational awareness

Reproduced with permission from Edozien, Leroy C. Towards safe practice in instrumental vaginal delivery. *Best Prac Clin Obstet Gynaecol*, 2007; **21**:639–55.

33 Trial of vaginal delivery after a previous caesarean section

All women with a uterine scar should have been assessed antenatally and a decision made as to mode of delivery (trial of vaginal delivery or elective CS). The guidance here applies only to a trial of vaginal delivery after one previous lower-segment CS.

Action plan for trial of vaginal delivery

- ☐ Inform the woman of the risk of scar rupture.
- ☐ Obtain IV access.
- ☐ FBC.
- ☐ Group-and-save.
- ☐ Monitor maternal pulse and BP.
- ☐ Set up continuous electronic fetal monitoring.
- ☐ Exclude malpresentation.
- ☐ Offer epidural analgesia.

Once labour is established, assess the cervix every 3 hours.

If the woman has not had a vaginal delivery previously, expect her progress to follow the pattern of a primipara.

A repeat of CS is indicated when the alert line on the partogram has been crossed by 2–3 hours.

Use of Syntocinon

- Syntocinon (oxytocin) should be used only with the approval of a senior obstetrician.
- It is relatively safe in the latent phase of labour, but high-risk if used to augment labour in the active phase.
- The woman must be informed of the increased risk of scar rupture. This discussion should be documented.
- Scar rupture is more likely to occur if prostaglandin has been given.
- Dose increments should be given at 30-minute intervals.
- Proceed to CS if there is no change in cervical dilatation 2 hours after commencement of Syntocinon infusion and good uterine action.
- Be extra vigilant for signs of imminent or actual scar rupture (see below): proceed to CS if any sign is observed.

Signs of scar rupture or imminent rupture

Things to look out for include:

- abnormal CTG (the most common sign)
- poor progress in labour
- sudden cessation of contractions
- reduction in intensity of contractions
- maternal tachycardia or hypotension
- shoulder tip or chest pain
- acute onset of tenderness at the CS scar site
- vaginal bleeding

If rupture is suspected then proceed to emergency CS.

> **!** Uterine rupture may occur without any warning signs.

Post-delivery

Transcervical palpation of the lower segment to exclude a scar rupture after vaginal delivery should not be performed routinely. It may be used to exclude a scar rupture if PPH occurs.

34 Induction of labour

The indication for induction and the patient's consent should be documented.

High-risk inductions should be commenced on the delivery suite.

Ideally, the woman would have been offered membrane-sweep before admission to the delivery suite and would have been informed that membrane-sweeping is not associated with increased risk of infection, but may cause discomfort and bleeding.

Methods

- **Prostaglandin E$_2$ (PGE$_2$, dinoprostone)**: if membranes are intact and the cervix is unfavourable (os closed or score < 7) for ARM.
- **ARM**: if the cervix is favourable and membranes are accessible.
- **Syntocinon (oxytocin) infusion**: if membranes are ruptured. If spontaneous rupture has not occurred, ARM should be performed before commencement of Syntocinon. Syntocinon infusion should not be started within 6 hours of the last dose of prostaglandin.

For all methods:

☐ Confirm indication and gestational age; obtain consent.
☐ Exclude contraindications:
  - major placenta praevia
  - abnormal lie.
☐ Commence CTG; if it is abnormal then inform the registrar.
☐ Perform cervical assessment:
  o cervical score (Table 34.1)
  o exclude cord presentation
  o proceed to ARM or prostaglandin induction.

Artificial rupture of fetal membranes

The midwife may perform ARM if the following criteria are met:

☐ The head is engaged.
☐ The vertex is presenting.
☐ Cord presentation has been excluded.

Table 34.1 Cervical score

	Score			
	0	1	2	3
Dilatation (cm)	<1	1–2	2–4	>4
Length (cm)	>4	2–4	1–2	<1
Consistency	Firm	Average	Soft	
Position	Posterior	Central	Anterior	
Station	−3	−2	−1 or 0	Below spines

Contraindications to ARM are:

- abnormal lie
- cord presentation
- placenta praevia

After ARM, check for cord prolapse and meconium staining of amniotic fluid. Document the fetal heart rate.

Prostaglandin induction of labour

- **Gel**: see the algorithms in Figures 34.1–34.3.
- **Tablets (intravaginal)**: dinoprostone 3 mg every 6–8 hours; maximum dose 6 mg for all women.

Use prostaglandin with caution in the following cases:

- previous CS
- multiple pregnancy
- breech presentation
- compromised fetus (IUGR, oligohydramnios, or abnormal CTG, Doppler ultrasound or biophysical profile)
- previous difficult labour or delivery
- grandmultipara
- asthma or glaucoma

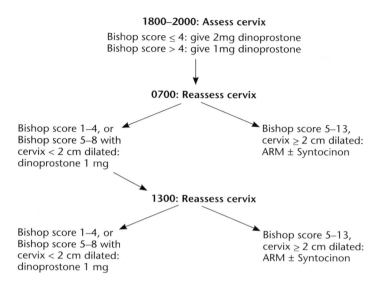

Figure 34.1 Algorithm for cervical ripening: nullipara.

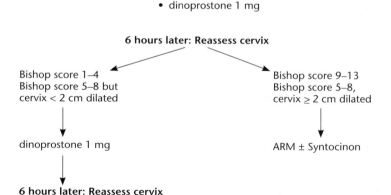

Figure 34.2 Algorithm for cervical ripening: multipara.

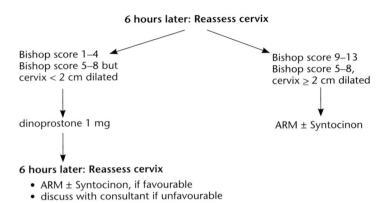

Figure 34.3 Algorithm for cervical ripening: previous caesarean section.

Monitoring following insertion of prostaglandin

☐ CTG monitoring: if normal, discontinue after 1 hour but continue intermittent auscultation.

☐ If uterine contractions have not started within the hour, the fetal heart rate should be recorded when contractions start.

☐ CTG should be done if the woman complains of abdominal or back pain.

☐ Maternal pulse, BP and contractions should be monitored half-hourly.

☐ The woman should remain in bed for 1 hour after administration of prostaglandin.

Precautions

• KY Jelly or chlorhexidine cream should not be used during administration of prostaglandin, since these delay absorption.

• Do not insert prostaglandin if you are unable to feel the cervix.

• Syntocinon should not be started within 6 hours of administering prostaglandin.

Hyperstimulation

In cases of hyperstimulation, administer tocolysis (see below).

Syntocinon infusion

Mix 10 units of Syntocinon in 500 mL compound sodium lactate (Hartmann's solution) or 0.9% saline, which gives a concentration of 20 milliunits/mL; with this dose, an infusion rate of 3 mL/h is equivalent to 1 milliunit/min.

Commence infusion at 2 milliunits/min (i.e. 6 mL/h); increase every 30 minutes until strong, regular uterine contractions – three in 10 minutes – are obtained.

A syringe driver or infusion pump must be used.

Do not exceed 32 milliunits/min (i.e. 96 mL/h); see Table 14.1.

Do not infuse through the same line as blood, plasma or insulin.

The syringe must be labelled, with the dose of drug and signatures of staff responsible on the label.

If labour is not established after 5 hours on this regimen then induction should be discontinued.

All women for whom labour is being induced with Syntocinon should have continuous electronic fetal monitoring.

A fluid balance chart should be kept.

The use of Syntocinon in the following circumstances requires the explicit approval of the consultant:

• multiple pregnancy
• malpresentation
• previous CS or other uterine scar
• grandmultiparity

Uterine hyperstimulation

This can occur with prostaglandin or Syntocinon.

Definition

• more than five contractions per 10-minute interval for at least 20 minutes (uterine tachysystole), or each uterine contraction lasting at least 2 minutes, or increased baseline uterine tone (uterine hypertonus)
• suspicious or pathological CTG

Management

This is the same procedure as augmentation with Syntocinon (see pp. 39–40).

35 Antenatal corticosteroid therapy

Indications

Corticosteroids should be given to women between 24 and 34 completed weeks' gestation presenting with any of the following:

- threatened preterm delivery
- APH
- preterm PROM
- any condition requiring elective preterm delivery

Note: Steroids may be given for this indication up to 36 weeks' gestation, but after 34 weeks, 94 women will need to be treated to prevent 1 case of respiratory distress syndrome.

Dose

Betamethasone 12 mg IM, two doses given 24 hours apart. (If delivery is likely to occur within 24 hours, the second dose may be given after 12 hours.)

Contraindications

Corticosteroids should not be given if there are any of the following:

- clinical evidence of chorioamnionitis (see p. 208)
- uncontrolled diabetes mellitus (see Chapter 52)
- tuberculosis
- porphyria

Beta-sympathomimetics

The combination of steroids and a beta-sympathomimetic tocolytic poses a risk of pulmonary oedema. When this combination is used, IV fluids should be kept to a minimum and a strict fluid balance should be kept. Observe the woman for chest pain, dyspnoea and cough, and discontinue the tocolytic therapy if any of these occur. Blood glucose and U/E should be checked every 6 hours.

Repeated doses

Repeated doses of prophylactic steroids should not be given.

Consider the possibility of adrenal insufficiency if a woman or baby who has been exposed to repeated doses of antenatal corticosteroids has an unexplained collapse.

36 Preterm prelabour rupture of membranes

This is the loss of amniotic fluid from the vagina before 37 weeks in the absence of uterine contractions. For management of PROM at term, see Chapter 10.

Action plan

☐ Perform a sterile speculum examination to confirm the diagnosis and exclude a prolapsed cord. Digital examination is not required unless the woman is in labour.

☐ Take swabs from the vagina (bacteriology) and endocervix (*Chlamydia*).

☐ FBC and group-and-save.

☐ Obtain a midstream specimen of urine.

☐ Perform an ultrasound scan for presentation, fetal growth and amniotic fluid volume.

☐ Liaise with the paediatrician.

Conservative management is indicated if infection is excluded and the woman is not in labour.

Delivery is indicated if any of the following occur:

- maternal pyrexia
- fetal tachycardia
- uterine tenderness
- meconium staining of amniotic fluid
- elevated CRP and/or leukocytosis (note that steroids may elevate the white cell count)
- offensive amniotic fluid
- gestation reaches 37 weeks

Conservative management

- Alert the neonatal unit.
- Give antibiotics after initial vaginal examination:
  - erythromycin 250 mg three times daily for 10 days
  - **do not give co-amoxiclav,** since this is associated with an increased risk of necrotizing enterocolitis in the newborn.
- Give betamethasone 12 mg IM, two doses 24 hours apart if gestation < 34 weeks.

- Take temperature and pulse rate 4-hourly.
- Monitor fetal heart rate daily.
- FBC and CRP twice-weekly.
- Perform an ultrasound/Doppler scan weekly (for amniotic fluid volume and fetal breathing movement).
- Scan fortnightly for fetal growth.

Mode of delivery, in the absence of other complications

- **Cephalic presentation**: vaginal delivery.
- **Breech presentation**: discuss with the woman and her partner the risks and benefits of CS versus vaginal delivery.

Induction of labour

- Syntocinon (oxytocin) infusion: see Table 14.1 for regimen.
- Prostaglandin may be used to ripen an unfavourable cervix (see p. 100 and Figures 34.1–34.3) and induce labour after preterm PROM, but:
  - o insert during a sterile vaginal examination
  - o use only one dose.

Labour

- ☐ Continue monitoring for signs of infection (temperature and pulse).
- ☐ Inform the paediatrician.
- ☐ Screen the baby for sepsis.

37 Preterm uterine contractions

Diagnosis

☐ Regular contractions (at least one every 10 minutes).
☐ Progressive cervical effacement and/or dilatation.
☐ Less than 37 completed weeks of gestation.

Action plan

☐ Confirm gestational age.
☐ Assess for symptoms of urinary tract infection.
☐ Assess for physical or emotional trauma.
☐ Check temperature and pulse.
☐ Check for uterine tenderness (consider placental abruption and chorioamnionitis).
☐ Assess frequency and duration of contractions.
☐ Assess fetal lie, presentation and station.
☐ Perform a speculum examination (exclude rupture of membranes), vaginal swab and endocervical swab.
☐ Assess the cervix.
☐ Obtain a midstream specimen of urine.
☐ FBC.
☐ U/E.
☐ Perform a Kleihauer test if the mother is Rh-negative.
☐ CTG.
☐ If there are <34 completed weeks, give corticosteroid: beta-methasone 12 mg IM, two doses 24 hours apart. **Steroids should not be used if there is clinical chorioamnionitis and should be used with caution in women with diabetes** (see p. 153).
☐ Inform the consultant obstetrician.
☐ Determine the underlying cause if possible.
☐ Consider transfer to a tertiary centre (see the guidelines for in utero transfer, p. 13).
☐ Decide (with the consultant) which of the following management options is to be followed:
  • suppression of labour (but see the contraindications below)
  • allow progression to vaginal delivery (see below)
  • CS, if indicated
  • observation, if the diagnosis of preterm labour is uncertain.

☐ Discuss with the parents regarding prognosis and management.
☐ Inform the paediatrician and neonatal unit.

Management of established preterm labour (when it is too late to suppress labour)

☐ Institute continuous electronic fetal monitoring.
☐ Avoid narcotic analgesia.
☐ Avoid FBS if <34 weeks.
☐ Avoid vacuum-assisted if <34 weeks.
☐ Alert paediatrician/SCBU (paediatric team to be present at delivery).
☐ Episiotomy is indicated if there is delay due to the head pushing against a tight perineum.
☐ Do not use 'prophylactic' forceps.

See also management of the pre-viable fetus (Chapter 38) and management of preterm breech presentation (Chapter 43).

There is no evidence to justify the routine use of prophylactic antibiotics for preterm labour with intact membranes.

Suppression of labour

Aims

• To enable the use of steroids for accelerating lung maturity.
• To allow in utero transfer, if necessary.

Options

• nifedipine (unlicensed for use in preterm labour)
• indomethacin (unlicensed)
• atosiban (licensed)
• magnesium sulphate ($MgSO_4$) (unlicensed)

Nifedipine is effective in suppressing preterm labour and has fewer side-effects and better neonatal outcome (lower incidence of jaundice, RDS and intraventricular haemorrhage).

Indomethacin is also effective, but is associated with premature closure of the fetal ductus arteriosus. This is more common in fetuses >32 weeks and where indomethacin has been administered for >48 hours.

Atosiban has significantly fewer maternal and fetal adverse effects. However, it is substantially more expensive.

> **!** A pragmatic approach is to use nifedipine or indomethacin initially. If the response is inadequate then a combination of both may be used. If response remains poor, or if contractions recur, then use atosiban.

Contraindications to suppression of labour

Do not attempt to suppress labour if any of the following apply:

- gestational age >35 weeks
- cervix >4 cm dilated
- signs/symptoms of chorioamnionitis
- abnormal CTG
- IUGR
- placental abruption
- bleeding (other than spotting) from placenta praevia
- hypertension/pre-eclampsia
- maternal thyroid or cardiac disease
- intrauterine fetal death
- fetal abnormality not compatible with survival

> **!** Before administering a tocolytic, exclude medical contraindications to the drug.

Nifedipine

Note: Do not use with magnesium sulphate or in women with significant cardiac disease.

As the use of nifedipine for preterm labour is off-label, it should be used strictly according to the local protocol.

Preload with 500 mL compound sodium lactate (Hartmann's solution) – because nifedipine is a calcium channel blocker and therefore lowers BP.

Loading dose

10 mg sublingually (the woman bites into the capsule and holds the liquid under her tongue). Repeat every 15 minutes until uterine contractions cease, up to a maximum dose of 40 mg (four capsules).

Maintenance dose

This is commenced 6 hours after the loading dose. The maintenance dose is dependent on the response to initial treatment:

- **If contractions stopped after 10 mg**: give 20 mg three times daily for 2–3 days.
- **If contractions stopped after 20 mg**: give 20 mg four times daily for 2–3 days.
- **If contractions stopped after 30 mg**: give 40 mg three times daily for 2–3 days.
- **If contractions stopped (or are still present) after 40 mg**: give 40 mg four times daily for 2–3 days.

Side effects: headache, palpitations, nausea, tachycardia.

Indomethacin (prostaglandins synthetase inhibitor)

Give 100 mg rectally as an initial dose, followed by 50 mg orally every 6 hours for 48 hours.

Do not use indomethacin if the gestational age > 32 weeks (it may cause premature closure of the ductus arteriosus) or if there is maternal or fetal renal disease, or severe oligohydramnios. If therapy continues beyond 48 hours, scan for amniotic fluid volume (it could cause digohydramnios as a result of reduced renal blood flow). Indomethacin is also contraindicated where there is a history of peptic ulcers or allergies to NSAIDs. It inhibits platelet aggregation, so should be used with caution in cases of APH or bleeding problems.

Side effects: (rare) headache.

Atosiban

Loading bolus

Give 6.75 mg IV as a bolus over 1 minute:

- Take a vial of atosiban 7.5 mg/mL and draw 0.9 mL; this contains the required loading dose of 6.75 mg.

Loading infusion

Give 18 mg/h IV for 3 hours.

Maintenance dose

Give 6 mg/h IV for 3–45 hours:

- Take two 5 mL vials each containing atosiban 7.5 mg/mL concentrate. Withdraw 10 mL from a 100 mL bag of 0.9% saline, leaving 90 mL. Add the contents of the atosiban vials to the 90 mL saline. This gives a solution of atosiban 75 mg/100 mL. Infuse this at 24 mL/h for 3 hours (loading infusion), then reduce to 8 mL/h Maintenance infusion).

The infusion is discontinued about 6 hours after contractions have ceased. The duration of treatment should not exceed 48 hours.

Side-effects include nausea, vomiting, headache and tachycardia.

Magnesium Sulphate

Check FBC, U&G, reflexes and urine output before commencing $MgSO_4$ tocolysis.

Loading dose

4g IV over 20 minutes (see p. 150).

Maintenance dose

1g/hour (see p. 150), for more than 48 hours.

Side effects: flushings, headaches, drowsiness. May cause respiratory depression in the neonate.

Symptoms of toxicity: respiratory depression, diminished or absent tendon reflexes (see p. 151).

☐ Monitor fluid input/output strictly.
☐ Check U/E after 24 hours.

Watch for pulmonary oedema, which may occur rapidly. Risk factors for this complication include iatrogenic fluid overload, multiple pregnancy, concomitant use of corticosteroid and infection.

Monitoring

Women on tocolytic drugs should be closely monitored:

- CTG
- frequency and strength of contractions
- side-effects of medication

Clinical judgement should determine whether or not further cervical assessment is required following administration of a tocolytic. Unecessary vaginal examination should be avoided.

38 Deliveries at the lower margin of viability

Pregnancy under 22 weeks

☐ The following points should be discussed and documented:
- Only 1 in 100 babies will survive, and of these half will have a severe disability.
- Delivery may be rapid.
- The baby may be born alive, move and/or gasp.

☐ Document the agreed management plan in the case notes.

Regardless of gestational age, if a baby shows any sign of life after delivery but subsequently dies, it should be registered as a live birth and neonatal death.

Pregnancy over 22 weeks

☐ The following points should be discussed and documented:
- The baby may survive short-term.
- Delivery may be rapid.

☐ A paediatrician and the SCBU must be informed.

☐ Give the parents an information leaflet about the very premature baby.

☐ Document the agreed management plan in the case notes.

A paediatrician should attend any birth after 20 weeks' gestation, because:

- The baby may be born alive.
- There may have been an error in assessment of gestational age.
- A decision not to resuscitate should be made by a paediatrician, not by an obstetrician or midwife.

> **!** If the woman wishes to use the toilet, the midwife should be alert. It is not uncommon for the small baby to be delivered in the toilet.

Post-delivery care if the baby does not survive

☐ Inform the consultant obstetrician of the birth.

- [ ] Agree postnatal care according to the wishes of the parents, and inform the GP, consultant obstetrician and community midwife.
- [ ] Inform the antenatal clinic and parent education coordinator.
- [ ] Offer post-delivery support, e.g. a link with the support group (see below).
- [ ] Inform the woman of the potential benefits of the recommended tests and investigations, and instigate as appropriate.
- [ ] Offer keepsakes and photographs.
- [ ] Discuss funeral arrangements and issue necessary documentation.
- [ ] Offer the opportunity to take the baby home before the funeral, and make necessary arrangements with the funeral director.

> **!** All live births must be registered, regardless of gestational age.

Support group

Sands (Stillbirth & Neonatal Death Charity)
    28 Portland Place
    London
    W1B 1LY

Helpline: 020 7436 5881 (0930 to 1730, Monday to Friday)
Office: 020 7436 7940 (1000 to 1700, Monday to Friday)
Fax: 020 7436 3715
Website: www.uk-sands.org

39 Multiple pregnancy

Triplets and higher-order pregnancies are normally delivered by elective CS. If the woman presents with uterine contractions then the consultant should be informed immediately, and a decision will be taken regarding the timing of delivery, depending on the frequency and strength of contractions. If the woman is in established labour then arrangements should be started for an urgent CS.

The following guidelines apply to the management of **twin pregnancies.**

First stage of labour

- [ ] The plan of management should be stated clearly antenatally; look for the plan in the case notes.
- [ ] On admission in labour:
  - Inform the registrar and anaesthetist.
  - Secure IV access.
  - FBC and group-and-save.
  - Set up continuous electronic monitoring of both twins (dual monitor).
- [ ] Recommend epidural analgesia.
- [ ] Examine lie/presentation of both twins, with the aid of an ultrasound scan:
  - **If both twins are cephalic**, proceed as with normal vaginal delivery.
  - **If the first twin is cephalic and the second twin non-cephalic**, anticipate normal delivery of the first twin, with possible recourse to CS if there are problems with the second twin.
  - **If the first twin is non-cephalic**, recommend CS.
- [ ] Prepare two neonatal resuscitation units.

> **!** Ensure that the CTG monitor is recording the heart rates of both twins, not a duplication of one twin's heart rate – be suspicious if the two traces are identical (or appear to be). Where there is doubt, application of a scalp electrode to the leading twin may be helpful.

Syntocinon (oxytocin) may be used to augment contractions, but this must be discussed first with a senior obstetrician.

Possible scenarios in the second stage should be discussed early in labour, so that the mother can prepare her mind for what may happen, e.g. delivery in theatre and manoeuvres to deliver the second twin. This is particularly important if the presentation of the second twin is non-cephalic, since the risk of having a CS after normal delivery of the first twin is (in the author's own experience) approximately 1 in 9. If the presentation of the second twin is non-cephalic then delivery should be conducted in theatre; alternatively, it could be conducted in an adjacent room, with regional anaesthesia and the theatre team primed.

Second stage of labour

- [ ] The following should be present: an experienced obstetrician, a paediatrician, two midwives and an anaesthetist.
- [ ] While the leading twin is being delivered, an assistant should attempt to stabilize the lie of the second twin.
- [ ] Record the time of delivery of the first twin. **Do not give Syntometrine** (ergometrine with oxytocin).
- [ ] Ensure that the umbilical cord is clamped properly (this is important in the case of shared fetal circulation). Use an additional clamp or marked clamps to distinguish the cords of the twins.
- [ ] Confirm the lie and presentation of the second twin by ultrasound scan.
- [ ] Perform a pelvic examination to assess presentation and descent.

Delivery of the second twin

Continue CTG monitoring. As long as the trace is normal, there is no reason to be worried about the clock, but CTG abnormalities are common when 30 minutes have elapsed.

Cephalic presentation

Confirm that the presenting part is in the pelvis. It will commonly be necessary to hold the baby's head over the pelvic brim. Perform ARM with the next uterine contraction, taking care to exclude cord presentation.

If there is a delay in re-establishing uterine contractions, start Syntocinon infusion: 10 units in 500 mL 0.9% saline or compound sodium lactate (Hartmann's solution); commence at 6 mL/h and double the rate every 5 minutes.

If uncomplicated vertex delivery is imminent, the midwife can deliver.

Breech presentation

- Offer ECV. If ECV is accepted and is successful then proceed as described above for cephalic presentation. If a Syntocinon infusion is running, it should be discontinued to facilitate ECV. It may be necessary to relax the uterus with IV glyceryl trinitrate or SC terbutaline.
- If ECV is declined or is attempted unsuccessfully then assisted breech delivery should be conducted by the obstetrician or a midwife skilled in the conduct of breech delivery.
- Before rupturing the membranes, ensure that the presenting part is in the pelvis – it will usually be necessary to hold the breech over the pelvic brim.
- Where ECV and assisted breech delivery are both declined, CS will have to be performed.
- In cases of footling breech, the options are breech extraction and CS.

Lie not longitudinal

The options are:

- Internal podalic version: grasp a foot vaginally through intact membranes, pull it down gently, and then perform ARM. An assisted breech delivery is then accomplished. This should always be performed in theatre.
- ECV, then proceed as described above for cephalic presentation.

If the above fail, or in the absence of an obstetrician skilled in podalic version, then resort to CS rather than try anything heroic.

Internal podalic version and breech extraction

The indications are:

- transverse lie
- failed ECV
- fetal distress

Do not attempt this if the membranes have ruptured.

The uterus should be well-relaxed; do not perform during a contraction, and discontinue Syntocinon infusion if one has been running. If necessary, IV glyceryl trinitrate (100 µg repeated at 2-minute intervals) or SC terbutaline 0.25 mg may be given to relax the uterus.

Preferably both feet of the baby should be grasped if breech extraction rather than assisted breech delivery is intended. If only one foot can be reached, this should be the anterior foot; if the posterior foot has been grasped, it should be rotated 180° to make it anterior – this is to avoid having the anterior buttock wedged astride the symphysis pubes.

Beware not to pull down an arm instead of the legs. The heel distinguishes a foot from a hand. Do not bring down a foot until the heel has been identified.

'I cannot emphasise too strongly that there is a world of difference between assisted breech delivery and breech extraction. The first necessitates only a series of simple manipulations with minimal analgesic or anaesthetic requirements. The second is – or can be – a formidable operation, with considerable danger to the fetus, and one which requires the help of full anaesthesia or major nerve-blocking procedures. Many a fetus is lost because an inexperienced medical attendant plunges into the second line of treatment when the conditions and preparations are suitable only for the first.'

Myerscough PR. *Munro Kerr's Operative Obstetrics*, 10th edn. London: Baillière Tindall, 1982: 76

Third stage of labour

☐ Active management should be used in the third stage – physiological management is contraindicated.

☐ Administer a Syntocinon infusion, 40 units in 500 mL for 4 hours.

☐ Perform a full examination of the placenta and membranes.

☐ If the twins are of the same sex, send the placenta for histological examination (to confirm chorionicity).

Indications for CS for second twin

- Acute fetal distress with vaginal delivery not imminent.
- Failure of the second twin to descend into the pelvis.
- Transverse lie with failed external version.
- Maternal haemorrhage, with vaginal delivery not imminent.
- Obstetrician not skilled in internal podalic version or breech extraction.

40 Abnormal lie in labour

This can be transverse or oblique.

- ☐ Exclude placenta praevia, ovarian cyst, uterine fibroids and other possible causes.
- ☐ CTG.
- ☐ Inform the woman of the risk of cord prolapse.
- ☐ Vaginal examination:
  - exclude cord presentation
  - assess the cervix
  - exclude ruptured membranes.

Intact membranes

- If there are no contraindications then discuss ECV (see Chapter 44).
- If ECV is declined or is attempted unsuccessfully then proceed to CS.
- Following successful version, consider ARM (in theatre) plus Syntocinon (oxytocin).

Ruptured membranes

- Avoid external version.
- Exclude arm prolapse.
- Deliver by CS.

Caesarean section

Obtain consent for 'caesarean section', not 'lower-segment caesarean section'.

Check before the operation whether the fetal back is inferior or superior:

- If the back is superior then it is easy to reach for the baby's legs and proceed with breech delivery, but beware that an arm may protrude from the uterine incision (put it back) or may be mistaken for a foot (look for the heel).
- If the back is inferior then internal version will usually be required, and the breech is usually easier to bring down than the head.

Difficult cases

For a preterm baby with the back inferior, a low vertical uterine incision should be considered.

For transverse lie with arm prolapse, a classical CS should be considered. If a transverse incision is used then this will almost always be converted to a J-incision and/or the baby will suffer a traumatic delivery. If a transverse incision is used then additional measures – such as relaxing or distending the uterus – should be employed (see below)

In some cases, it may be necessary to relax the uterus to facilitate delivery of the baby. This can be achieved with SC terbutaline 0.25 µg or IV glyceryl trinitrate 100 µg.

Uterodistension

For difficult cases **where the fetal membranes have ruptured**, the author devised the technique of uterodistension to facilitate lower-segment CS delivery. These cases include transverse lie with arm prolapse and early preterm delivery with longitudinal lie and ruptured membranes, where a classical incision would otherwise be indicated.

In this technique, 500–1000 mL of warm (room temperature) 0.9% saline is infused via a giving set inserted into the uterine cavity through a stab (1.0 cm) incision in the lower pole of the uterus. Pressure on the bag of fluid is required. Once the cavity is sufficiently distended, the incision is extended and the baby is delivered. This technique allows the use of a low incision where a classical (upper-segment) incision would otherwise have been necessary.

41 Occipitoposterior position

This should be suspected if:

- The baby's back is difficult to feel.
- Fetal heart tones are heard better towards the flank.
- There is significant back pain.

Confirm by vaginal examination.

To ensure rotation of the head, good uterine activity is required, so consider the use of Syntocinon (oxytocin) if the frequency and strength of contractions are suboptimal, particularly in a nulliparous woman. This also reduces the chances of a prolonged labour.

Hands-and-knees maternal posture may influence fetal position.

Persistent occipitoposterior position

The options for effecting vaginal delivery are:

- vacuum-assisted delivery, with posterior cup
- Kjelland's forceps delivery
- manual rotation:
  - lithotomy position (or left lateral)
  - adequate analgesia

Ensure that the criteria for instrumental delivery are met before proceeding with forceps or ventouse.

Nulliparity and occipitoposterior position carry a high risk of injury to the anal sphincter complex, so an episiotomy is recommended.

In skilled hands, the Kiwi OmniCup vacuum device is as good as Kjelland's forceps in effecting rotation, as well as less traumatic to the mother.

42 Malpresentation

The baby's presentation reflects the degree of flexion or extension of the head:

- full flexion: occiput
- full extension: face
- deflexed but not fully extended: brow

☐ Inform the registrar or senior obstetrician.
☐ Group-and-save.
☐ Rule out fetal abnormalities (anencephaly, goitre and hydocephalus).

Brow presentation

The forehead is the presenting part palpable on vaginal examination. Frontal sutures, anterior fontanelle, orbital ridges, eyes and the root of the nose are palpable.

This may change to a face or vertex presentation, and so, if the woman is in early labour, await events. If there is slow progress or secondary arrest, proceed to CS. If diagnosed in advanced labour then CS is indicated.

Face presentation

This is diagnosed by palpation of the chin, mouth, nose and orbital ridges. It may be mistaken for a breech presentation.

If the woman is in early labour and cephalo-pelvic disproportion has been excluded, allow to progress.

If the woman is in advanced labour, check whether the position is mentoanterior or mentoposterior:

- If it is mentoanterior then vaginal delivery is feasible; allow to progress, proceeding to CS if progress is poor. An episiotomy will usually be required.
- If it is mentoposterior then vaginal delivery is not feasible, but there is a one in four chance of rotation on reaching the pelvic floor, so you may wait and see; if the position is persistently mentoposterior then perform CS.

Where vaginal delivery is anticipated, inform the mother in advance that the baby's face may be temporarily swollen (oedema) and this may cause initial difficulties with feeding.

If there are CTG abnormalities then proceed to CS. Note that FBS is contraindicated.

At CS, flex and rotate the head to occipitotransverse before delivery.

Compound presentation

This could be a cephalic presentation with a foot or hand palpable or a breech presentation with a hand palpable (take care to distinguish between hand and foot).

Manage as normal for a cephalic or breech presentation, unless there is cord prolapse.

43 Breech presentation

Breech presentation may be diagnosed antenatally or in labour.

For cases diagnosed antenatally, the mode of delivery should be stated clearly in the antenatal records.

Vaginal delivery should be performed only by a skilled attendant.

Undiagnosed breech in labour

☐ Confirm the presentation by ultrasound scan.
☐ Determine the wishes of the mother regarding mode of delivery.
☐ If the membranes are intact, assess suitability for ECV (see Chapter 44).
☐ Recommend CS if any of the following occur:
  • pelvis clinically small or anatomically abnormal
  • placenta praevia
  • big baby (consider parity and the weight of previous babies delivered vaginally)
  • hyperextended fetal head
  • footling presentation
  • IUGR
  • previous perinatal death
  • bad obstetric history
  • medical problems or other risk factors.
☐ The mode of delivery should always be discussed with the consultant.

Preterm breech in labour

☐ Inform the consultant.
☐ Offer epidural analgesia (which prevents pushing before full cervical dilatation).

There is insufficient evidence to justify routine CS for preterm breech. The decision regarding mode of delivery should be made after full discussion with the woman (and her partner, if present). The discussion should be documented.

Breech vaginal delivery

First stage of labour

- ☐ Discuss the risks of breech vaginal delivery.
- ☐ Discuss epidural analgesia (which prevents pushing before full cervical dilatation and facilitates delivery, but may inhibit pushing in the second stage).
- ☐ Institute continuous electronic fetal monitoring. A monitoring electrode may be applied to the buttock if an abdominal transducer is not giving a good trace.
- ☐ Obtain IV access: FBC and group-and-save.
- ☐ The anaesthetist must be available immediately.
- ☐ Alert the paediatrician.
- ☐ Explain the delivery to the woman and partner/relative (involving the latter is important, since they will observe the delivery).
- ☐ ARM is performed only if the presenting part is applied well to the cervix.
- ☐ Perform a vaginal examination immediately after spontaneous rupture of membranes (to exclude cord prolapse).
- ☐ Following spontaneous or artificial rupture of membranes, observe the CTG closely for the first 10 minutes (because of the risk of occult cord prolapse).
- ☐ Give oral ranitidine 150 mg.
- ☐ Poor progress despite good contractions suggests that the pelvis is inadequate.
- ☐ Augmentation is not contraindicated. However, discuss with the consultant before using a Syntocinon (oxytocin) infusion. **Do not use Syntocinon if there is secondary uterine inertia**.
- ☐ FBS from the buttock may be performed if fetal distress is suspected – but the only published study suggesting reliability of fetal buttock blood sampling was based on 10 cases only.

Second stage of labour

> **!** Consider CS if there is delay in the second stage.

- ☐ If the woman has not had an epidural then delivery is better conducted in theatre, with the patient prepared for an emergency general anaesthetic.

- ☐ Delivery should be conducted by an experienced obstetrician or appropriately trained midwife.
- ☐ An anaesthetist and a paediatrician should be present.
- ☐ The woman should be placed in the lithotomy position and catheterized.

Allow the breech to descend spontaneously. This is an assisted vaginal delivery, not a breech extraction, so traction should be avoided. Traction could result in extension of the arm and the head, making delivery more difficult.

Unless the perineum is relaxed, perform an episiotomy when the fetal anus is seen over the fourchette. Use a pudendal block if there is no epidural.

The fetal spine usually rotates uppermost. If the legs are extended then deliver them by flexion at the knee joint and abduction/extension at the hips

Encourage the mother to push out the breech until the scapulae are visible.

- Cover the baby with a towel.
- Pull down a loop of cord only if necessary.
- Hold the femurs with your thumbs on the sacrum and your other fingers on the anterior superior iliac crest (pelvifemoral grip), avoiding any pressure on the fetal abdomen.
- Run your finger over the shoulder and down to the elbow to deliver the arm.
- If the arms are extended, gently rotate one shoulder anteriorly and bring the arm down across the chest (Lovset's manoeuvre). The nuchal line should now be visible.

Delivery of the head

You must see the nape of the neck before proceeding with delivery of the head.

- After an assistant has gently lifted the leg almost to the vertical, deliver with forceps. **Caution**: doing this prematurely could hyperextend the neck and cause damage to the cervical spinal cord.
- Use the Mauriceau–Smellie–Veit manoeuvre if delivery is imminent and there is no time to apply forceps.
- If the head fails to engage, the baby may be allowed to hang for up to 1 minute until the nuchal line is visible (Burns–Marshall

technique). Suprapubic pressure can also be applied to guide the head into the pelvis.

Arrest of the after-coming head

This may be due either to entrapment behind an incompletely dilated cervix or to arrest at the pelvic brim. If the cervix not fully dilated then incise it at the 4 and/or 8 o'clock positions, taking care not to cut the baby.

For arrest at the pelvic brim, apply suprapubic pressure and/or McRoberts manoeuvre (flexion and abduction of the hips).

Caesarean section for breech presentation (elective or emergency)

Confirm by ultrasound in theatre that the presentation is still breech.

Take care with opening the uterus – scalpel injuries to the baby are more likely to happen in breech than cephalic presentation. A good-size uterine incision is required, particularly in preterm deliveries, to prevent entrapment and traumatic delivery of the baby's head.

44 External cephalic version

External cephalic version (ECV) should be offered to all women with a breech presentation, provided that the following apply:

- Gestational age ≥ 37 weeks.
- There is no contraindication to ECV.
- There is no indication for CS.

Risks of ECV

- cord accidents
- feta-maternal transfusion
- placental abruption
- rupture of uterus or uterine scar

Contraindications to ECV

- ruptured membranes
- vaginal bleeding
- abnormal CTG
- Rh isoimmunization
- uterine malformation
- previous myomectomy
- placenta praevia
- multiple pregnancy

Cautions

ECV may be performed in the following circumstances, but the mother should be informed of the increased risks:

- previous CS
- previous episode of bleeding
- IUGR
- oligohydramnios
- obesity
- pre-eclampsia

Action plan

- ☐ Provide an information leaflet.
- ☐ Obtain consent.
- ☐ Perform an ultrasound scan to confirm lie and presentation, assess amniotic fluid volume and exclude placenta praevia.
- ☐ Perform CTG for 20 minutes before ECV.
- ☐ Give a tocolytic: terbutaline 0.25 mg SC about 15 minutes before ECV.
- ☐ Make no more than three attempts at ECV, over 5 minutes.
- ☐ After ECV, perform an ultrasound scan to confirm presentation.
- ☐ Perform CTG for at least 20 minutes after ECV.
- ☐ If the woman is Rh-negative, send a blood sample for a Kleihauer test and give anti-D immunoglobulin 500 units (unless the baby's father is also Rh-negative).
- ☐ Proceed to CS if the CTG is abnormal or if the procedure has provoked vaginal bleeding.
- ☐ Document CTG observations, tocolytic given, outcome of procedure and further care.
- ☐ Agree a follow-up plan:
  - **If ECV is successful**, follow up in the antenatal clinic.
  - **If ECV is unsuccessful**, proceed to elective CS or breech vaginal delivery; document the mother's/couple's decision.

If a woman has had a successful ECV, she should be monitored closely in labour, since there is a higher incidence of CS for various reasons.

45 The woman with genital mutilation

Check the notes for any special instructions.
Anticipate problems and discuss these with the woman:

- difficult vaginal examination
- difficulty in catheterizing the bladder
- difficulty in applying an FSE (if required)
- genital tract trauma during delivery
- possible need for an anterior midline episiotomy
- psychological distress
- post-delivery urinary retention (due to pain)
- vulvovaginal haematoma

Respect the woman's views and cultural identity, and try not to sound patronizing.

Action plan

☐ Offer epidural analgesia: this will facilitate vaginal examination and de-infibulation.
☐ If vaginal examination is difficult or impossible, the cervix may be assessed by rectal examination, but specific consent for this must be obtained.
☐ An episiotomy will probably be necessary; this will often be a midline anterior episiotomy in cases of infibulation.
☐ Provide psychological support postpartum. This may require referral to psychosexual services.

> **!** Restoring infibulation (stitching together of the labia) after delivery is illegal under the Female Genital Mutilation Act 2003.

If the baby is female and the family supports female circumcision, social services should be informed. Explain to the woman why this is necessary. Alert the health visitor to possible child-protection issues.

Female Genital Mutilation Act 2003

- A person is guilty of an offence if he excises, infibulates or otherwise mutilates the whole or any part of a girl's labia majora, labia minora or clitoris.
- A person is guilty of an offence if he aids, abets, counsels or procures a girl to excise, infibulate or otherwise mutilate the whole or any part of her own labia majora, labia minora or clitoris.
- The law permits a registered doctor or midwife to perform a surgical operation on a girl who is in any stage of labour, or has just given birth, for purposes connected with the labour or birth. This in practice means the woman can be de-infibulated but not re-infibulated.

46 The obese woman in labour

With obese women (BMI >40):

- The possibility of missing abnormalities on scans is higher.
- Monitoring the baby in labour is more difficult.
- Siting epidurals is difficult.
- Surgery is more difficult.
- There is a risk of thromboembolism.
- Breastfeeding is important to help postnatal weight loss.
- Preventative management of pressure sores is important.
- A larger operating theatre table is required.

☐ Alert SpR and anaesthetist.
☐ Check for any care plan devised antenatally.
☐ Use an appropriate size sphygmomanometer cuff to measure BP.
☐ Secure venous access as early as possible.
☐ Consider insertion of arterial line, especially if pre-eclamptic.
☐ Group-and-save (increased risk of PPH).
☐ VTE prophylaxis per protocol.
☐ Anticipate shoulder dystocia.
☐ Senior obstetrician to be present if CS is required and BMI is >40.

47 Perineal tear

The perineum should be inspected after every delivery, and the presence or absence of any tear should be documented.

Classification of perineal tears

- **First degree**: laceration of vaginal epithelium or perineal skin only.
- **Second degree**: also injury to perineal muscles, but not the anal sphincter.
- **Third degree**: disruption of vaginal epithelium, perineal skin, perineal body and anal sphincter muscles:
    - **3a:** involving <50% of the thickness of the external sphincter
    - **3b:** involving >50% of the thickness of the external sphincter; complete tear of the external sphincter
    - **3c:** internal sphincter torn as well
- **Fourth degree**: torn anal sphincter and rectal mucosa.

All tears extending to the anal margin should be regarded as third-degree tears until proven otherwise.

First- and second-degree tears: episiotomy

See also Chapter 25.

Vaginal tears and episiotomies should be repaired with 2/0 Vicryl Rapide.

Infiltrate with 1% lidocaine, not exceeding 20 mL.

Care should be taken to start the repair from the apex of the tear.

For skin closure, a continuous subcuticular suture is associated with less short-term pain than interrupted sutures. Apposing but not suturing the skin is associated with less dyspareunia.

A paravaginal haematoma should be suspected if there are signs of shock after the third stage of labour in the absence of significant bleeding externally. See also Chapter 78.

☐ A rectal examination should be performed after the repair.
☐ A swab and needle count should be performed after the repair.
☐ If there is a substantial periurethral tear then insert a catheter.

Third- and fourth-degree tears

Repair must be performed by an obstetrician trained to do so and must be performed in the operating theatre.

> **!** A general anaesthetic or epidural/spinal is mandatory when there is a third- or fourth-degree tear.

- [ ] The anal epithelium should be repaired with Vicryl 3/0 (Ethicon) sutures, either interrupted with the knots tied in the anal lumen or continuous submucosal.
- [ ] The internal anal sphincter should be repaired with 3/0 PDS (Ethicon) interrupted sutures.
- [ ] The external anal sphincter should be repaired with 3/0 PDS sutures, using either overlapping or end-to-end technique. A systematic review of three randomized controlled trials concluded that compared to immediate primary end-to-end repair, early primary overlap repair 'appears to be associated with lower risks for faecal urgency and anal incontinence symptoms'. However, the experience of the surgeon was not addressed in the three trials (see Further reading).
- [ ] Vaginal repair should be done using Vicryl Rapide.
- [ ] Reconstruct the perineal muscles (failure to do so leaves a short, deficient perineum).
- [ ] Skin repair should be done using Vicryl Rapide.
- [ ] A swab and needle count should be performed after the repair.
- [ ] Give cefuroxime 1.5 g and metronidazole 500 mg IV, followed by a 5-day course of oral cefalexin and metronidazole.
- [ ] Prescribe:
  - lactulose 10 mL three times daily for 2 weeks
  - Fybogel, one sachet twice daily for 2 weeks.
- [ ] Document the extent of injury and how it was managed. The use of a repair proforma is recommended.
- [ ] Arrange a follow-up appointment with a consultant obstetrician and/or perineum clinic, according to the local protocol.

48 Heart disease in labour

Principles of management

Delivery must be planned, particularly for women with severe heart disease. Liaison between consultant obstetrician, anaesthetist and cardiologist is essential. In most cases, vaginal delivery is preferred to CS.

Prevent heart failure – avoid factors that may increase cardiac workload, including:

- excessive physical effort – use epidural analgesia and prophylactic instrumental delivery
- anaemia
- infection
- hypertension

In women with obscure febrile illness, consider the possibility of endocarditis.

Action plan

☐ **Antibiotic cover**: all women in labour and with a structural heart defect, prosthetic valve or a history of endocarditis must have prophylactic antibiotics:
  - **CS**: amoxicillin 1 g IV and gentamicin 120 mg IV (over 3 minutes) at induction of anaesthesia, then amoxicillin 500 mg 6 hours later.
  - **Vaginal delivery**: amoxicillin 1 g IV and gentamicin 120 mg IV (over 3 minutes) at the onset of labour or ruptured membranes, then amoxicillin 500 mg 6 hours later.
  - **If the woman is allergic to penicillin or has had more than a single dose of penicillin in the previous month**: vancomycin 1 g by slow IV infusion (over at least 60 minutes) before delivery, then gentamicin 120 mg IV at induction of anaesthesia or at 8 cm dilatation.
☐ Labour should take place in the left lateral or upright position. Avoid supine hypotension.

- [ ] ECG.
- [ ] Administer oxygen by mask, as required.
- [ ] Institute continuous CTG.
- [ ] Offer epidural analgesia (take care with fluid preloading; avoid if cardiac output is restricted).
- [ ] Produce a fluid balance chart.
- [ ] Expedite the second stage of labour (elective forceps or ventouse).
- [ ] Give Syntocinon (oxytocin) by slow infusion for the third stage of labour (5 units in 500 mL at 125 mL/h). **Do not give ergometrine or Syntometrine (ergometrine with oxytocin)**.
- [ ] If PPH due to atony occurs, misoprostol 800 µg PR should be used instead of carboprost (Hemabate), since it is less vasoactive.
- [ ] Continue high-dependency care for 24–48 hours following delivery: the most dangerous time for the cardiac patient is the first 24 hours after delivery. Women with Eisenmenger's syndrome need to be in the ITU for at least 7 days after delivery.

Some women with cardiac disease will be taking anticoagulant medication such as warfarin or clopidogrel (a platelet antagonist). If the woman is on anticoagulants:

- Avoid IM injections.
- Involve the on-call haematologist.
- Stop anticoagulant at commencement of labour.
- Resume anticoagulants post-delivery if there is no PPH.

If labour starts while the patient is on warfarin, then vitamin K should be given to the mother and to the baby at delivery.

Preterm labour

Discuss with the consultant before commencing tocolytics.

Tocolytics, in particular nifedipine, may compromise cardiac function. Atosiban is the preferred tocolytic.

> **!** In patients with heart disease, avoid fluid overload and local anaesthetics containing adrenaline.

49 Peripartum cardiomyopathy

This is a disease of unknown cause in which left ventricular dysfunction occurs in late pregnancy or puerperium. The condition is rare before 36 weeks. It is characterized by the absence of recognizable heart disease before the last month of pregnancy and the absence of a known cause of heart failure.

Diagnosis

The above, plus left ventricular systolic dysfunction on echocardiography.

> **!** Any woman without a relevant prior history and who presents with heart failure in late pregnancy should be regarded as having a cardiomyopathy until it is proven otherwise.

Risk factors

- advanced age
- multiparity
- African descent
- hypertension
- multiple pregnancy

Symptoms and signs

- breathlessness
- palpitations
- swollen legs
- tachycardia
- dyspnoea
- dysrhythmia
- signs of embolism

Action plan

- ☐ **Call for help!**
- ☐ Manage shock: airways, breathing, circulation.
- ☐ Establish IV access.
- ☐ FBC, U/E and group-and-save.
- ☐ Chest X-ray.
- ☐ ECG.
- ☐ Echocardiography.
- ☐ Impose salt and water restriction.
- ☐ Institute continuous electronic fetal monitoring.
- ☐ Involve a cardiologist immediately.
- ☐ Inform a neonatologist.
- ☐ Inform an anaesthetist.
- ☐ Institute anticoagulant therapy and treatment of heart failure as agreed with the cardiologist.

A senior clinician must decide the place, time and mode of delivery. Transfer to a high-risk centre, if feasible.

50 Pre-eclampsia

Pre-eclampsia remains one of the main causes of maternal mortality and morbidity worldwide. It manifests as new hypertension ≥140/90 mmHg and proteinuria ≥2+ on dipstick analysis or >0.3 g/24 h, after 20 weeks' gestation. Women who become hypertensive and either have symptoms or have abnormal haematological or biochemical results should also be regarded as having pre-eclampsia until proven otherwise.

> **!** Not all cases present with the classic features.

Complications of pre-eclampsia include:
- cerebrovascular accident
- placental abruption
- HELLP syndrome
- DIC
- eclampsia
- hepatic failure
- renal failure
- pulmonary oedema
- IUGR

Pre-eclampsia is classified as severe if any of the following are seen:

- dizziness, drowsiness, visual symptoms, epigastric pain/tenderness or chest pain
- hyperreflexia
- papilloedema
- systolic BP > 160 mmHg or diastolic BP > 110 mmHg
- MAP > 125 mmHg
- proteinuria: 3+ on dipstick or >3 g in a 24-hour urine collection
- oliguria: <500 mL in 24 hours
- thrombocytopenia: <100 × 10^9/L
- creatinine > 100 mmol/L
- ALT > 50 IU/L
- pulmonary oedema

> 'Pre-eclampsia is a disease of signs ... symptoms are the hallmark of imminent eclampsia.'
>
> Baskett TF. *Essential Management of Obstetric Emergencies*, 3rd edn. Bristol: Clinical Press, 1999: 79

!
- Mild pre-eclampsia may progress rapidly to severe disease.
- Fits may occur without any warning signs or symptoms.
- Fits occur more frequently postpartum than intrapartum.

Action plan

- ☐ Check symptoms.
- ☐ Check reflexes and fundoscopy.
- ☐ Obtain a serial BP recording (see below).
- ☐ Perform a urinalysis.
- ☐ FBC.
- ☐ Group-and-save.
- ☐ U/E and creatinine.
- ☐ Urate.
- ☐ LFT.
- ☐ Perform a clotting screen.
- ☐ Insert a 16G Venflon: Hartmann's solution 85 mL/h.
- ☐ Monitor urine output.
- ☐ Offer epidural analgesia if platelet count $> 100 \times 10^9$/L.
- ☐ Institute continuous electronic fetal monitoring.
- ☐ Inform consultant obstetrician.
- ☐ Inform the consultant anaesthetist.
- ☐ Assess fetal wellbeing: growth, amniotic fluid volume and umbilical artery Doppler ultrasound.
- ☐ Decide whether to deliver or manage conservatively. This generally entails an evaluation of risks and benefits, but the following is a useful guide:
  - **severe pre-eclampsia**: deliver, regardless of gestational age
  - **mild/moderate pre-eclampsia at term**: deliver
  - **mild/moderate pre-eclampsia preterm**: may be managed conservatively.

☐ If delivery is imminent, give ranitidine 150 mg orally immediately, then 150 mg every 6 hours.
☐ If <34 weeks' gestation, give prophylactic betamethasone for lung maturity.
☐ Commence antihypertensive treatment (see below).

Measurement of blood pressure

Automated BP-monitoring devices are convenient for monitoring trends, but they may underestimate BP. If a device is used, the readings must be checked hourly against sphygmomanometer measurements.

The sphygmomanometer cuff should be at the level of the heart, and should be of an appropriate size for the woman. In women whose arm circumference exceeds 35 cm, a large cuff should be used.

Korotkoff sound V (disappearance of the sound) should be used for determining diastolic pressure, not Korotkov IV (muffling).

Severe pre-eclampsia

☐ Manage in a quiet room.
☐ Open a high-dependency care chart.
☐ Connect an ECG monitor.
☐ Connect an O_2 saturation monitor. If O_2 saturation drops below 95%, inform the registrar.
☐ Record BP every 15 minutes; when it is stable, this can be done hourly.
☐ Check the respiratory rate hourly.
☐ Document the EWS
☐ Insert a Foley catheter, and monitor fluid balance (see p. 146).
☐ Commence anticonvulsant prophylaxis (see below).
☐ Consider insertion of an arterial line. An arterial line can be used as an adjunct to non-invasive BP monitoring, particularly in obese women and when there has been a major haemorrhage.
☐ Consider insertion of a CVP line if there is excessive bleeding at delivery and in cases of placental abruption. If CVP < 5 cmH_2O or > 12 cmH_2O then inform the anaesthetist.
☐ Consider insertion of an arterial line. This facilitates precise and continuous monitoring of BP.
☐ If epidural analgesia is accepted, avoid fluid load.
☐ CTG.
☐ If delivery is not imminent, perform an ultrasound scan for fetal growth, amniotic fluid volume and Doppler assessment.

> **!** Do not transfer to another hospital unless the woman's clinical condition has been stabilized. Her BP should be below 160/105 mmHg and her oxygen saturation should be normal. (See also in utero transfer, p. 13.)

Delivery

Timing

Timing of delivery should be judicious. Stabilizing the patient before CS will reduce risks, but delaying delivery could increase risks; each case should be assessed on its merits.

Second stage of labour

If the active phase lasts beyond 30 minutes, advise instrumental delivery.

Third stage of labour

Give Syntocinon (oxytocin) 5 units IV or IM. **Do not use ergometrine or Syntometrine (ergometrine with oxytocin).**

Watch for PPH

Note that with haemoconcentration, pre-eclamptic patients are less tolerant of haemorrhage than normotensive women: observe BP and urine output.

Post-delivery

- Avoid NSAIDs (e.g. diclofenac).
- Manage on the delivery suite until stable.
- Maintain vigilance.
- Check BP hourly for the first 4 hours, then every 4 hours for 12 hours, and then every 8 hours for 48 hours.
- Continue antihypertensive and anticonvulsant treatment as required (see below).
- Give thromboembolism prophylaxis (see p. 169).

Antihypertensive therapy in pre-eclampsia

The aim of treatment is not to normalize BP but to maintain it at a relatively safe level. If BP drops too low, placental perfusion will be reduced. This is particularly stressful to the growth-restricted fetus. Aim for a MAP < 125 mmHg.

- **If systolic BP < 160 mmHg, or diastolic BP < 105 mmHg, or MAP is in the range 125–140 mmHg**, give oral labetalol 200 mg. Expect BP to drop within 30 minutes.
- **If systolic BP > 160 mmHg, or diastolic BP > 105 mmHg, or MAP > 140 mmHg**, the options are hydralazine or labetalol. Hydralazine is more widely used and was described as 'the first-line drug of choice for management of severe hypertension' (*Why Mothers Die. Report on Confidential Enquiries into Maternal Deaths in the UK, 1994–96*. London: The Stationery Office, 1998: 92). Meta-analyses have not shown one drug to be clearly superior to another. In the author's experience, hydralazine is particularly helpful in women of African descent who are not responsive to labetalol.

Labetalol

☐ Give 200 mg orally, if the woman is able to tolerate oral therapy, or a bolus of 50 mg (10 mL labetalol 5 mg/mL) IV over 10 minutes. This may be repeated at 15-minute intervals up to a maximum of four doses (i.e. 200 mg).

☐ Follow with a labetalol infusion 5 mg/mL delivered via a syringe pump at a rate of 4 mL/h (20 g/h). Double the rate every 30 minutes until BP is stable and within the target range. The maximum dose is 32 mL/h (160 mg/h).

Side-effects of labetalol include headache, postural hypotension (avoid an upright position for 3 hours after IV labetalol) and nausea.

Contraindications to labetalol

- severe asthma or obstructive airways disease
- heart block
- severe peripheral arterial disease

Hydralazine

- [ ] Give hydralazine 5 mg bolus IV over 10 minutes.
- [ ] Simultaneously give 500 mL Gelofusine (or other colloid) over 30 minutes (see p. 148).
- [ ] If required, follow with a hydralazine infusion 40 mg in 40 mL 0.9% saline, via a syringe pump, starting at 5 mL/h.
- [ ] Titrate against BP as follows: double every 30 minutes until stable at a diastolic BP of 90 mmHg or the pulse rate exceeds 130 beats/min; do not exceed 40 mL/h.

Side-effects of hydralazine include tachycardia, headache, dizziness, dyspnoea and flushing. These mimic deteriorating pre-eclampsia.

> **!** Do not use hydralazine in women with cardiovascular disease.

When tailing off hydralazine (this is usually post-delivery), halve the infusion rate every 30 minutes.

Anticonvulsant prophylaxis in pre-eclampsia

All women with severe pre-eclampsia should receive anticonvulsant prophylaxis.

Loading dose: 4 g

- [ ] Take one ampoule of 5 g (ml) magnesium sulphate (MgSO₄), and draw 8 ml. Dilute this with 22 ml of 5% dextrose.
- [ ] Administer via a syringe pump over 10 minutes (i.e. infusion rate of 180 ml/hour).

Warning: a bolus given too rapidly may cause cardiac arrest.

Maintenance dose: 1 g/hour

- [ ] Take two ampoules of 5 g MgSO₄ and dilute in 30 ml of 5% dextrose. This gives a solution of 1 g/5 ml. Infuse via a syringe driven at 5 ml per hour.

Review hourly to ensure that:

- respiratory rate > 12/min
- urine output > 20 mL/h

- knee or forearm jerk is present
- O_2 saturation $\geq$ 95% on air or oxygen

Check serum magnesium level 4 hours after commencing infusion.
If reflexes or respiration are depressed, stop $MgSO_4$ infusion and check the serum magnesium level. See below for management of magnesium toxicity.
If urine output < 20 but > 10 mL/h then adjust treatment according to the plasma creatinine level:

- **Normal creatinine (100 mmol/L)**: continue infusion but check the magnesium level every 2 hours.
- **High creatinine (100–150 mmol/L)**: reduce infusion to 0.5 g/h and check the magnesium level every 2 hours.
- **Very high plasma creatinine (>150 mmol/L)**: stop $MgSO_4$ infusion. Check the magnesium level at once and every 2 hours thereafter.

If urine output < 10 mL/h, stop $MgSO_4$ infusion.

Magnesium sulphate blood levels

- **Therapeutic**: 2–3.5 mmol/L.
- **Low**: <2 mmol/L. Increase the infusion rate to 2 g/h for 2 hours, then recheck level.
- **High**: 3.5–5.0 mmol/L. Stop infusion. Restart at half the previous rate if urine output > 20 mL/h.
- **Very high**: >5.0 mmol/L. Stop infusion. Commence ECG.

Management of magnesium toxicity
Features

- loss of deep tendon reflexes
- nausea
- double vision
- slurred speech
- respiratory arrest
- cardiac arrhythmia
- cardiac arrest (in severe cases)

If magnesium toxicity is suspected:

☐ Discontinue $MgSO_4$ infusion.
☐ Check magnesium level urgently.

☐ ECG.
☐ If cardiorespiratory arrest is imminent, give 10% calcium gluconate 10 mL IV over 2–5 minutes.
☐ **If cardiac arrest occurs, crash call and cardio-pulmonary resuscitation.**

Postpartum

Continue MgSO$_4$ for 24 hours postpartum, or longer if the woman is still hyperreflexic. If MgSO$_4$ was commenced post-delivery, continue for 24 hours.

Continue antihypertensives until diastolic BP < 100 mmHg or MAP < 125 mmHg.

Post-delivery ward round (days 0–3)

It is important for doctors and midwives to remain alert after delivery, since some women may suffer a postnatal deterioration.

☐ Check temperature, pulse, BP and respiratory rate. Chart EWS.
☐ Check O$_2$ saturation. If O$_2$ saturation < 95% or respiratory rate > 25/min, request a chest X-ray.
☐ Assess sensorium. Abnormal sensorium with hyperreflexia is indicative of cerebral oedema.
☐ Check fluid balance.
☐ Exclude abnormal bleeding.
☐ FBC and coagulation screen every 8 hours for the first 24 hours.
☐ LFT daily.
☐ Suspect hepatic rupture if right upper quadrant pain is persistent: arrange a CT scan.
☐ Medication: do current doses of antihypertensive and other medication need to be adjusted?

Fluid management in pre-eclampsia

Principles

Problems related to excessive fluids (pulmonary oedema and ARDS) are much more common than those related to inadequate fluids. ARDS is the most frequent mode of death from hypertensive disorders of pregnancy.

In severe pre-eclampsia, there is an increase in systemic vascular resistance. Vasodilator therapy can reduce this, resulting in precipitate hypotension and poor end-organ perfusion. Vasodilator therapy should therefore be accompanied by a fluid load to maintain or improve organ (placenta and kidneys) perfusion.

In severe pre-eclampsia, BP may be maintained despite regional blockade. Preloading with fluids (before epidural) in anticipation of hypotension may be an unnecessary risk in this situation.

Oedema mobilizes back into the circulation within 24–36 hours after delivery.

Patients with excessive haemorrhage require totally different management, including invasive monitoring in many cases.

Pre-delivery

- Background fluids: Hartmann's solution 85 mL/h.
- If Syntocinon infusion has been given, the volume should be included in the calculation of fluid input. **Note**: if a woman with severe pre-eclampsia requires a Syntocinon infusion, a high concentration (30 units in 500 mL 0.9% saline) should be used (Table 49.1).
- Correct any pre-existing fluid deficits (due e.g. to a long period of nil by mouth, vomiting or blood loss).
- Maintain a strict fluid input/urine output chart.

Table 49.1 Syntocinon infusion regimen for women with severe pre-eclampsia

Time after starting (min)	Amount of Syntocinon infused (milliunits/min)	Volume infused (mL/h)
0	2	2
30	4	4
60	8	8
90	12	12
120	16	16
150	20	20
180	24	24
210	28	28
240	32	32

- Give a fluid bolus of 500 mL Gelofusine or Haemaccel over 30 minutes before or at the same time as:
  - loading with magnesium sulphate
  - loading with an antihypertensive drug

or if urine output < 100 mL in 4 hours.

> **!** Do not give any woman more than two fluid boluses, unless she is bleeding.

> **!** Diuretics (e.g. furosemide 10–20 mg) are not appropriate except in pulmonary oedema.

Delivery is indicated if there is:

- pulmonary oedema
- renal failure (rising urea/creatinine)
- irreversible oliguria despite the above measures

Post-delivery

- Ensure that peripartum losses have been replaced. Note that a natural diuresis occurs postpartum.
- Background fluids: Hartmann's solution 50 mL/h for 24 hours, then 85 mL/h. Total fluid input in the first 24 hours should not exceed 2 L.
- Replace any continuing loss. Check U/E (watch for hyponatraemia).
- Look for signs of pulmonary oedema: rising respiratory rate and heart rate, O_2 saturation < 95% on air, chest signs and abnormal chest X-ray. If present, give furosemide as above, whatever the urine output. Also give oxygen.
- CVP monitoring will usually be required in patients with significant haemorrhage, renal failure or pulmonary oedema that does not respond rapidly to normal therapeutic measures.

Management of oliguria (<80 mL in 4 hours)

- **If the woman is hypovolaemic (see below) or bleeding,** replace loss.

- **If the woman is not hypovolaemic (see below) and not bleeding:**
  - Provided that there are no signs of fluid overload and that fluid input in the last 24 hours has not exceeded output by >750 mL, give 200 mL IV fluid (colloid) over 30 minutes. If urine output does not improve, give furosemide 10 mg IV.
  - If fluid input exceeds output by >750 ml, do not give colloid infusion; give furosemide 10 mg IV.
  - If oliguria persists, consult a renal physician.

Features of hypovolaemia

- dry mouth
- loss of skin turgor
- cold extremities
- raised pulse rate
- hypotension
- reduced pulse pressure
- raised respiratory rate

> **!** Tachypnoea could also be a sign of fluid overload (pulmonary oedema).

Blood transfusion

Blood transfusion may increase the intravascular oncotic pressure and cause pulmonary oedema in a woman with severe pre-eclampsia. Unless it is absolutely necessary (e.g. acute blood loss), transfusion should be withheld until after diuresis has occurred.

51 Eclampsia

Management aims to:

- control convulsions
- control BP
- deliver the baby

Beware of postpartum eclampsia (see below).

Action plan

☐ Maintain the airway.
☐ Turn the patient to the left lateral position.
☐ Administer oxygen by mask (at least 10 L/min).
☐ Insert an IV line.
☐ Arrest convulsions with $MgSO_4$. Diazepam 10 mg IV may also be used.
☐ Prevent further fits with $MgSO_4$ infusion.
☐ Treat hypertension.

Anticonvulsant treatment (magnesium sulphate)

Loading dose: 4 g

☐ Take one ampoule of 5 g (ml) magnesium sulphate ($MgSO_4$), and draw 8 ml. Dilute this with 22 ml of 5% dextrose.
☐ Administer via a syringe pump over 10 minutes (i.e. infusion rate of 180 ml/hour).

Warning: a bolus given too rapidly may cause cardiac arrest.

Maintenance dose: 1 g/hour

☐ Take two ampoules of 5 g $MgSO_4$ and dilute in 30 ml of 5% dextrose. This gives a solution of 1 g/5 ml. Infuse via a syringe driven at 5 ml per hour.

Review hourly to ensure that:

- respiratory rate > 12/min
- urine output > 20 mL/h
- knee or forearm jerk is present
- O_2 saturation ≥ 95%

> **!** If convulsions recur, give 2 g (10 mL) 20% MgSO$_4$ solution over 5 minutes.

The maintenance dose should be continued for 24 hours after the last seizure.

Side-effects of MgSO$_4$ infusion include double vision, slurred speech, respiratory depression, loss of tendon reflexes, cardiac arrhythmia and cardiac arrest.

If reflexes or respiration are depressed, stop MgSO$_4$ infusion and check serum magnesium level. Respiratory depression should be treated with calcium gluconate 1 g (**10 mL** of **10%** calcium gluconate) IV given over **10 minutes**.

If urine output < 20 but > 10 mL/h, adjust treatment according to the plasma creatinine level:

- **Normal creatinine (100 mmol/L)**: continue infusion but check the magnesium level every 2 hours.
- **High creatinine (100–150 mmol/L)**: reduce infusion to 0.5 g/h and check the magnesium level every 2 hours.
- **Very high plasma creatinine (>150 mmol/L)**: stop MgSO$_4$ infusion. Check magnesium level at once and every 2 hours thereafter.

If urine output < 10 mL/h, stop MgSO$_4$ infusion (MgSO$_4$ is mostly excreted in urine, so oliguria could be associated with toxicity).

Magnesium sulphate blood levels

- **Therapeutic**: 2–3.5 mmol/L.
- **Low**: <2 mmol/L. Increase the infusion rate to 2 g/h for 2 hours, then recheck level.
- **High**: 3.5–5 mmol/L. Stop infusion. Restart at half the previous rate if urine output > 20 mL/h.
- **Very high**: >5 mmol/L. Stop infusion. Commence ECG.

Persistent seizures

If seizures persist despite magnesium:

- Try diazepam 10 mg IV.
- An anaesthetist may give thiopentone 50 mg IV.
- Consider intubating the patient.

- Further seizures should be managed by intermittent positive-pressure ventilation and muscle relaxation.
- If the fits are refractory, a CT or MRI scan should be performed.

Controlling blood pressure

This is as for management of hypertension in pre-eclmpsia (p. 143).
Avoid a precipitous drop in BP.

General management

This is as for pre-eclampsia (Chapter 50).

- A decision must be made immediately regarding mode of delivery.
- After delivery, the woman should remain in HDU until at least 24 hours have elapsed without a fit.
- Anticonvulsant therapy should be continued until 24 hours have elapsed since the last fit and the woman is no longer hyperreflexic.
- Fluid management is as for pre-eclampsia (p. 146).

> **!** If there are focal neurological signs then CT or MRI scan of the brain should be performed.

> **!** One woman had a seizure in hospital after a CS for pre-eclampsia at term and appeared to be making a good recovery, but was found collapsed and pulseless after being left unattended in a bath on the fourth day after delivery.
>
> *Why Mothers Die. Report on Confidential Enquiries into Maternal Deaths in the UK, 1994–96.* London: The Stationery Office, 1998: 39

52 Diabetes mellitus

Management will depend on whether the woman is on insulin.

Details of intrapartum management will usually have been decided in the joint diabetic clinic and written in the case notes.

Induction of labour or CS in a diabetic woman should be performed first thing in the morning.

Induction of labour by artificial rupture of fetal membranes

- The woman should have her usual dose of insulin the evening before.
- She should be nil by mouth from midnight.
- At 0800, perform ARM and commence insulin/glucose protocol (see below).

Induction of labour with prostaglandin

- Allow the patient to eat and drink.
- The woman should have her usual dose of insulin until she is in established labour.
- Commence insulin/glucose protocol when she is in established labour.

Elective caesarean section

- The woman should have a bedtime snack the night before, then nil by mouth.
- She should have her usual evening dose of insulin, or as prescribed by the diabetologist.
- The morning dose of insulin should be skipped.
- CS should be performed in the morning (first on the list).
- A sliding scale of insulin should be given in theatre (women with gestational diabetes are unlikely to need this).

First stage of labour

☐ Institute continuous fetal monitoring.
☐ Recommend epidural analgesia.
☐ FBC, U/E, group-and-save.

- ☐ Check urine for ketones.
- ☐ Insert two IV lines:
  - **Line 1**: 5% glucose + 10 mmol KCl 500 mL at 100 mL/h through an infusion pump (for a pre-eclamptic patient on fluid restriction, use 10% glucose at 40 mL/h).
  - **Line 2**: 0.9% saline 50 mL + short-acting insulin 50 units (i.e. a concentration of 1 unit/mL), via a pump according to a sliding scale (Table 51.1) (for a pre-eclamptic patient on fluid restriction, use 25 units in 50 mL).
- ☐ Check capillary blood glucose hourly. The meter used for capillary blood glucose measurement should be checked by comparing a capillary reading with the value obtained for a venous sample sent to the laboratory – the readings should not differ by more than 1.0 mmol/L.

Aim to keep the blood glucose concentration in the range 4–7 mmol/L.

- If blood glucose is below this range, give glucose (e.g. 60 mL Lucozade, 100 mL Ribena or IV 10% glucose 150 mL) and recheck blood glucose.
- If blood glucose falls outside this range 3 hours after starting the sliding scale, call the diabetologist.

Use separate IV access for IV Syntocinon (oxytocin) or preloading for epidural.

The infusion pump and lines should be checked every hour. **Be cautious with the use of a three-way tap for glucose/**

Table 51.1 Sliding scale for insulin infusion

Blood glucose concentration (mmol/L)	Insulin infusion rate (units/h)
≤2	0
2.1–3.9	0.5
4.0–6.9	1
7.0–8.9	2
9.0–10.9	4
11.0–16	6
>16	8

insulin infusions, since inadvertent disconnection of one line could be disastrous.

> **!** Always check that the glucose drip is working.

If there are difficulties with blood glucose control, check the following:

- The pump may not be working.
- The glucose drip may not be working or may be running into tissue.
- Syntocinon may have been added to glucose instead of to saline.

> **!** If Syntocinon is required, it should be via saline infusion, not glucose.

Beware of secondary arrest, in view of possible macrosomia.
  If shoulder dystocia is anticipated:

- Discuss this with the woman.
- Revise the shoulder dystocia drill now.

Gestational diabetes, diet-controlled

☐ Check blood glucose on admission and then hourly:
  - **If blood glucose <3.9 mmol/L or labour lasts >8 hours**, commence dextrose 5% infusion.
  - **If blood glucose >7 mmol/L**, commence insulin/glucose protocol (see above). Insulin may be needed in the second stage of labour owing to a catecholamine surge.
☐ On the day after delivery, check blood glucose levels: preprandial, 2 hours after lunch and at bedtime.
☐ Arrange a glucose tolerance test at 6–8 weeks post-delivery.

Preterm labour

See also Chapters 36 and 37.
  Manage according to the diabetic protocol.
  Ritodrine should not be used.

Betamethasone may affect blood glucose control – so avoid if glucose control on admission is poor. If glucose control on admission is satisfactory, the effect of dexamethasone can be controlled by increasing the dose of SC insulin in consultation with the diabetologist (see p. 104).

After delivery

Perform capillary blood glucose monitoring every 2 hours.

Gestational diabetes

- Discontinue insulin/glucose infusion once the woman is able to eat a light diet.
- She may eat and drink a normal diet without SC insulin.

Type 1 and type 2 diabetes

- Once the placenta is delivered, reduce the insulin dose by 50%.
- Continue the sliding-scale infusion until the woman is able to eat and drink.
- The first SC dose of insulin should overlap the IV infusion by 30 minutes.
- Monitor blood glucose pre-meal and at bedtime
- Restart SC insulin on the pre-pregnancy dose. If this is not known, seek advice from the diabetologist.
- If the woman was on oral hypoglycaemic agents prior to her pregnancy, check whether this is compatible with breastfeeding.

Do not transfer to the postnatal ward until blood glucose levels are normal and there is no ketonuria.

Hypoglycaemic shock

> **!** **Call for help**: anaesthetist and Specialty Trainee in medicine.

Do a quick dipstick test to determine whether this is hypoglycaemia (<2.5 mmol/L) or ketoacidosis (usually, but not always, >9 mmol/L).

Manage shock: airways, breathing, circulation.

- [ ] Institute continuous electronic fetal monitoring.
- [ ] Give 50 mL of 50% glucose IV.
- [ ] Chart vital signs and O_2 saturation.
- [ ] Repeat finger-prick glucose every 30 minutes.

Diabetic ketoacidosis

Risk factors include infection, stress, and the use of steroids to accelerate fetal lung maturity.

Presentation

- nausea
- vomiting
- polydipsia
- dizziness
- air hunger
- tachycardia
- tachypnoea
- hypotension
- smell of ketones

> **! Call for help**: anaesthetist and Specialty Trainee in medicine.

The woman needs high-dependency or intensive care. The consultant anaesthetist and diabetologist should be engaged in the management of this condition.

Do a quick dipstick glucose test to confirm that this is ketoacidosis (usually, but not always, >9 mmol/L), rather than hypoglycaemia (<2.5 mmol/L).

Manage shock: airways, breathing, circulation.

- [ ] Institute continuous electronic fetal monitoring.
- [ ] Chart vital signs and O_2 saturation.
- [ ] Blood tests: FBC, glucose, U/E, group-and-save, blood culture and arterial blood gases.
- [ ] Obtain a midstream specimen of urine for bacteriology.
- [ ] Urinalysis.
- [ ] Insert a Foley catheter: monitor fluid input and urine output.
- [ ] Insert a nasogastric tube (to reduce the risk of aspiration).
- [ ] Treat dehydration: IV infusion of 0.9% saline.

- ☐ Check capillary blood glucose hourly.
- ☐ Administer insulin as advised by the physician (usually a loading dose of 10 units insulin, followed by an infusion of 5–10 units/h).
- ☐ Give 20–40 mmol of potassium in each litre of 0.9% saline, over 3 hours.
- ☐ Treat infection, if present.
- ☐ If the woman is undelivered, determine the time and mode of delivery.
- ☐ Alert the paediatricians.

53 Asthma (acute exacerbation in labour)

Women with well-controlled asthma usually have healthy pregnancies, normal labour and good perinatal outcomes and should be advised to continue their usual asthma medication in labour. Acute exacerbation of asthma in labour is rare, but should be treated aggressively when it occurs. It can be precipitated by stress, medication (see below) or upper respiratory tract infection.

Drugs that can cause or aggravate bronchospasm

- ergometrine
- NSAIDs (e.g. diclofenac)
- beta-blockers (e.g. labetalol)
- prostaglandin F_2 analogues (carboprost/Hemabate)

Note: prostaglandin F_2 and oxytocin are safe.

Action points

☐ Document pulse rate, respiratory rate and EWS: respiratory rate > 25/min and pulse rate > 110 beats/min are consistent with exacerbation.

☐ Record oxygen saturation.

☐ Check peak expiratory flow (PEF). This is a measure of how fast the patient can breathe out (exhale) air: it is the amount of air that she can forcibly blow out in 1 second, measured in litres. PEF < 50% of predicted normal is consistent with severe exacerbation.

☐ Chest X-ray.

☐ FBC.

☐ U/E.

☐ Arterial blood gas analysis:
- hypercapnia: $PaCO_2$ > 6 kPa
- hypoxia: PaO_2 < 8 kPa
- acidosis

If any of the above occur then repeat the test 30–60 minutes after commencement of treatment.

☐ Administer oxygen to achieve an O_2 saturation ≥ 95%.

☐ CTG.
☐ Exclude differential diagnoses: pulmonary embolism (PE), pulmonary oedema, cardiac disease and aspiration.
☐ Avoid morphine; use fentanyl instead.
☐ Recommend epidural as it decreases oxygen consumption and reduces hyperventilation.
☐ Consult a medical specialist.
☐ Consider use of a bronchodilator.
☐ Consider a corticosteroid: inhaled, oral or IV prednisolone 30 mg orally or hydrocortisone 100 mg IV.

If there is no response to treatment then admission to the ICU is indicated.

Women who have used oral steroids for >2 weeks prior to delivery should be given hydrocortisone 100 mg IV every 8 hours to cover the stress of the labour. The reason for this is that theoretically the prolonged use of systemic steroids could suppress the hypothalamic–pituitary axis, with the result that the usual release of adrenal corticosteroids during labour does not occur and symptoms of adrenal insufficiency may be observed during or after delivery.

After delivery

• Breastfeeding is not contraindicated.
• Physiotherapy should be given.
• Administer salbutamol 2.5–5 mg via a nebulizer.
• In severe cases, consider an IV bronchodilator:
    o aminophylline 250 mg/30 min
    o salbutamol 200 µg/10 min
    o terbutaline 200 µg/10 min.

54 Epilepsy

Management in labour

- Reassure that most women with epilepsy will have a normal, vaginal delivery.
- Continue the usual anticonvulsant regimen during labour and postpartum. If vomiting occurs within 1 hour of ingestion, administer the same dose again.
- Discuss pain control. Pethidine is contraindicated since it is metabolized to norpethidine, which could trigger a fit.
- Inadequate analgesia induces hyperventilation (which could trigger a fit).
- Avoid exhaustion and dehydration – these may trigger fits. Fits may also be triggered by bright flickering lights, noise, lack of sleep and emotional stress.
- The woman must not be left on her own.
- If the woman has had a previous seizure in labour or is at increased risk of seizures (e.g. owing to stress or fear), she can be given oral clobazam 10 mg, two doses 12 hours apart.
- Give appropriate support in cases of congenital malformation or dysmorphic features.
- Check that resuscitation equipment is readily available.

Indications for caesarean section

- status epilepticus
- uncontrolled repeated seizures
- fetal distress

Management of fits in labour

- **Call for help**.
- Place the woman in a wedged position (to avoid vena cava compression).
- Keep her head lower than her body, to allow any vomit to drain.
- Clear her airways.
- Administer oxygen by facemask.
- Give IV lorazepam 4 mg bolus. If required, a further 1 mg bolus is given slowly. Use a large vein.

- Alternatively, give IV diazepam 10 mg; further 2 mg boluses may be given if required, but do not exceed a total of 20 mg. However, lorazepam is less sedative, and so associated with a lower risk of aspiration.
- If this fails to control seizures (i.e. the woman is in status epilepticus), give IV phenytoin 15 mg/kg at an infusion rate ≤ 50 mg/min.
- In status epilepticus, endotracheal intubation may be required.

Do not leave the woman unattended.

    Do not restrain her.

    Do not put anything in her mouth.

    Do not give her anything by mouth until you are certain that she is fully recovered.

After seizure

- Reassure the woman when she recovers.
- Make her comfortable (she may have had involuntary loss of urine during seizure).
- CTG.

If there is doubt whether a seizure in labour is due to eclampsia or epilepsy, then, in addition to IV lorazepam or diazepam, a slow IV bolus of 4 g magnesium sulphate over 5–10 minutes followed by 1 g/h for 24 hours is recommended.

After delivery

The mother needs sleep. Postnatal exhaustion and sleep deprivation may precipitate seizures. A short course of oral clobazam 10 mg nocte for 2–4 days can be given if necessary.

Vitamin K 1 mg should be given to the baby at birth if the mother has been using anticonvulsant medication.

Encourage breastfeeding, but support the woman in her choice of feeding method. Anticonvulsant drugs are excreted in breast milk in low concentrations, but the risks to the baby (irritability and lethargy) are minor compared with the benefits of breastfeeding. However, if the mother is on lamotrigine, warn her that the baby may have a skin rash, in which case breastfeeding will have to be discontinued.

> **!** Fits can occur in the immediate postnatal period, resulting in accidents to mother and baby.

Give advice regarding infant care to minimize danger to the baby in the event of the mother having a fit. Accidents can also occur during a bath or shower, so a midwife or health worker should be aware and the door should not be locked.

Review anticonvulsant medication and discuss contraception.

With the woman's consent, report to the UK Epilepsy and Pregnancy Register, Room 105, Bostock House, Royal Victoria Hospital, Grosvenor Road, Belfast BT12 6BA. Tel (free-of-charge): 0800 389 1248.

55 Systemic lupus erythematosus

Principles

Systemic lupus erythematosus (SLE) is an immunological disorder in which antibodies are formed against the body's own DNA and other cellular components. It is characterized by vasculitis and antinuclear antibodies. Other manifestations include cutaneous and neurological signs. The woman may present on the delivery suite with intrauterine fetal demise, pre-eclampsia, IUGR or preterm labour.

- Implement a plan agreed and documented antenatally.
- Watch for:
    o acute exacerbation in labour
    o hypertension
    o thrombosis
    o congenital heart block
    o neonatal lupus.
- Features of a flare include fever, arthralgia, myalgia, rash, oral ulcers and hypertension.

It may be difficult to distinguish lupus flare from pre-eclampsia. Also, pre-eclampsia may coexist with lupus flare. In lupus flare, urine microscopy shows red blood cells, leukocytes and granular casts.

- Transfer of antibodies across the placenta may result in congenital heart block.
- A paediatrician should be present at delivery.
- CS should be performed for obstetric indications.

Action plan

☐ Institute continuous electronic fetal monitoring.
☐ Check FBC, serum urate, creatinine, urea and electrolytes on admission.
☐ Urinalysis.
☐ Monitor hourly urine output.
☐ Alert an anaesthetist.
☐ Alert a paediatrician.
☐ Liaise with a rheumatologist and the immunology laboratory.

☐ If the woman is on long-term steroid therapy, give hydrocortisone 100 mg IV every 8 hours (three doses) because of inhibition of the pituitary–adrenal axis.

☐ If acute exacerbation occurs, discuss management with the medical team. Steroids may be required.

Neonatal lupus

This syndrome comprises congenital heart block, transient cutaneous lupus lesions and systemic manifestations. It occurs in 5% of babies born to women with SLE.

56 Other connective tissue disorders

> **!** If the woman is on long-term steroid therapy, give hydrocortisone 100 mg IV every 8 hours (three doses) because of inhibition of the pituitary–adrenal axis.

Rheumatoid arthritis
- If the woman has been on NSAIDs, watch for peripartum haemorrhage.
- Watch for pre-eclampsia.
- If woman is unable to fully abduct the hip, this may impede vaginal delivery.
- Rarely, atlanto-axial subluxation complicates general anaesthesia.
- Institute continuous electronic fetal monitoring.

Marfan syndrome
- Institute continuous electronic fetal monitoring.
- Check the notes for a plan agreed with the cardiologist.
- If aortic root diameter > 4 cm then recommend elective CS (because of the risk of aortic dissection).
- Vaginal delivery is possible in uncomplicated cases.
- If the woman has heart-valve incompetence, give prophylactic antibiotics (Chapter 72).

Ehlers–Danlos syndrome, types I–IX
These are inherited disorders of collagen metabolism, characterized by fragile skin and blood vessels and by hypermobility of the joints.

Women with types I and IV disease are more likely to develop complications in pregnancy, with a mortality rate of 20–25% in type IV disease. PROM occurs frequently.

Malpresentation in labour is common, and the baby may be growth-restricted.

Potential problems include rupture of the great vessels during labour, vaginal and perineal tears, rupture of the scar in women with previous CS, difficulties with intubation, PPH, delayed wound healing and genital prolapse.

The mode of delivery should be decided by the consultant in discussion with the woman.

SECTION 3
Haemorrhage and haematological disorders

57 The rhesus-negative woman

Approximately 60% of babies born to Rh(D)-negative women in the UK are Rh-positive. Sensitized Rh-negative women with a significant antibody titre will usually be transferred to a tertiary centre. The following applies to non-sensitized women.

Sensitizing events

Following any potentially sensitizing event, such as trauma, placental abruption, vaginal bleeding, external cephalic version (ECV) or amniocentesis:

- Give anti-D immunoglobulin 500–1000 units.
- Carry out a Kleihauer test, and then give additional anti-D if indicated.

At delivery

- The midwife who conducts delivery or receives the baby in theatre should obtain cord and maternal blood within 2 hours of delivery for a Kleihauer screening test.
- If unable to obtain cord blood, the midwife must perform a heel prick before the mother and baby are transferred to the postnatal ward.

All Rh-negative women who have given birth to a Rh-positive baby should be given anti-D within 72 hours of delivery.

Transfusions

If a Rh-negative woman receives a platelet transfusion, check the product to confirm whether it is Rh-positive or Rh-negative platelets. If it is Rh-positive then anti-D should be given (discuss with the haematologist).

If a Rh-negative woman receives Rh-positive blood in error, discontinue the transfusion immediately. Send a maternal blood specimen for estimation of the volume of Rh-positive cells in circulation. Give anti-D 500 units for every 4 mL of Rh-positive blood transfused. Refer to the local protocol for managing transfusion errors.

58 Thromboembolism prophylaxis

All women, irrespective of history, should have general measures (mobilization and avoidance of dehydration) to minimize the risk of VTE.

Specific thromboprophylaxis is indicated in:

- all patients undergoing CS
- women in normal labour and with a history of thrombosis, thrombophilia or other risk factors

Thromboprophylaxis for caesarean section

All women undergoing CS should be assessed for thromboembolism risk and given appropriate prophylaxis, depending on their risk category. A thromboembolism risk assessment proforma should be completed by the doctor obtaining consent for surgery.

Low risk

- elective CS
- uncomplicated pregnancy and no other risk factors

Prophylaxis

☐ thromboembolism-deterrent stockings (appropriate size and fitted correctly)
☐ early mobilization and hydration

Moderate risk

Women with any one of the following risk factors:

- age > 35 years
- obesity (>80 kg)
- parity ≥ 4
- gross varicose veins
- current infection
- pre-eclampsia
- immobility before surgery (>4 days)

- major current illness (e.g. heart or lung disease, cancer, inflammatory bowel disease, nephrotic syndrome, or sickle cell disease)
- emergency CS in labour
- excessive blood loss

Prophylaxis

☐ thromboembolism-deterrent stockings or intermittent pneumatic compression
☐ early mobilization and hydration
☐ dalteparin (Fragmin) 5000 units SC daily until discharge (other LMWH can be substituted)

High risk

- two or more risk factors from the above
- extended major pelvic or abdominal surgery (e.g. CS or hysterectomy)
- personal or family history of DVT, pulmonary embolism or thrombophilia
- paralysis of lower limbs
- antiphospholipid antibody (cardiolipin antibody or lupus anticoagulant)

Prophylaxis

☐ thromboembolism-deterrent stockings or pneumatic compression
☐ early mobilization and hydration
☐ dalteparin 5000 units SC daily until the fifth postoperative day, or until fully ambulant if longer
☐ continue with dalteparin or warfarin for 6 weeks post-delivery

The first dose of dalteparin should be given when the patient returns to the postnatal ward.

Thromboprophylaxis in vaginal deliveries

Many women requiring intrapartum thromboprophylaxis will have been identified antenatally. Some will have been commenced on heparin or aspirin earlier in pregnancy. Check the notes for the regimen prescribed. For others, assess the risk and institute prophylaxis as follows.

Low risk

- uncomplicated pregnancy

Prophylaxis

☐ early mobilization and hydration

Moderate risk

Women with any two of the following risk factors:

- age > 35 years
- obesity (>80 kg at booking)
- parity ≥ 4
- gross varicose veins
- current infection
- pre-eclampsia
- immobility before delivery (>4 days)
- major current illness (e.g. heart or lung disease, cancer, inflammatory bowel disease, nephrotic syndrome, or sickle cell disease
- labour ≥ 12 hours
- excessive blood loss

Prophylaxis

☐ early mobilization and hydration
☐ thromboembolism-deterrent stockings or pneumatic compression
☐ dalteparin 5000 units SC daily until discharge

High risk

- three or more risk factors from the above
- extended major pelvic or abdominal surgery (e.g. CS or hysterectomy)
- personal or family history of DVT, PE or thrombophilia
- paralysis of lower limbs
- antiphospholipid antibody (cardiolipin antibody or lupus anticoagulant)

Prophylaxis

- ☐ thromboembolism-deterrent stockings or pneumatic compression
- ☐ early mobilization and hydration
- ☐ dalteparin 5000 units SC daily until the fifth postoperative day, or until fully ambulant if longer
- ☐ continue with dalteparin or warfarin for 6 weeks post-delivery

Dalteparin injection should be commenced within 6 hours of delivery.

Regional analgesia

Discuss with the anaesthetist if epidural/spinal analgesia is planned (see also below).

Thrombin time should be checked before the administration of an epidural/spinal block.

> **!** Regional analgesia reduces the risk of DVT. General anaesthesia increases the risk of DVT.

> **!** Thromboembolism-deterrent stockings can be harmful if fitted incorrectly.

Regional analgesia and dalteparin

Insertion of spinal/epidural block

This must not be done until at least 12 hours after the last dose of dalteparin (this will apply mostly to women who have had antenatal prophylaxis).

Removal of epidural catheter

This must not be done until 12 hours after the last dose of dalteparin. After removal of the catheter, wait at least 6 hours before administering the next dose of dalteparin.

59 Acute venous thromboembolism and pulmonary embolism

Risk factors

- obesity
- immobility
- grandmultiparity
- previous DVT
- dehydration
- surgical procedures
- APH or PPH
- pre-eclampsia
- thrombophilia (see Chapter 63)
- age > 35 years
- infection
- operative delivery
- sickle cell disease
- inflammatory disorder
- long-distance travel

Clinical features

- leg pain, swelling or tenderness
- chest pain, breathlessness, haemoptysis
- faintness or collapse
- pyrexia
- raised jugular venous pressure

Initial investigations

- ☐ FBC
- ☐ U/E and LFT
- ☐ coagulation screen
- ☐ D-dimer
- ☐ thrombophilia screen (if starting on anticoagulant; see below)

Suspected DVT

☐   compression or duplex ultrasound scan

Suspected PE

☐   pulse oximetry
☐   arterial blood gases
☐   ECG
☐   chest X-ray
☐   V/Q scan
☐   Doppler ultrasound leg studies (bilateral)

Any woman with signs or symptoms suggestive of VTE should undergo diagnostic imaging to confirm or exclude the diagnosis.

> **!** The D-dimer test is a negative predictive test: a low level suggests that there is no VTE, but a high level may be normal in pregnancy.

If it is not possible to perform diagnostic imaging on the same day then treatment should be initiated while awaiting objective diagnosis, unless treatment is strongly contraindicated.
If an ultrasound scan for DVT is negative but clinical suspicion is high then continue anticoagulant treatment and request a venogram.

Management

• See the algorithms shown in Figures 59.1 and 59.2.
• Consult a haematologist.
• Apply graduated elastic compression stockings.
• Administer anticoagulant treatment (see below).
• For DVT, measure leg circumference daily.
• Encourage ambulation.

Anticoagulant therapy for DVT and PE

The woman should be screened for thrombophilia before anticoagulant therapy is commenced.

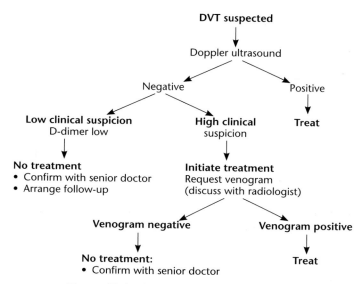

Figure 59.1 Algorithm for suspected DVT.

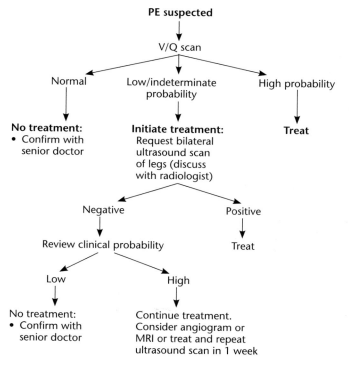

Figure 59.2 Algorithm for suspected PE.

Thrombophilia screen

(This comprises two EDTA bottles plus three citrate bottles. Indicate the gestational age on the card.)

- anticardiolipin antibodies
- lupus anticoagulant
- protein C
- protein S
- activated protein C resistance
- factor V Leiden mutation
- prothrombin G20210A mutation

As levels of some of these factors vary in pregnancy, the results should be interpreted in consultation with the haematologist.

Low-molecular-weight heparin (LMWH)

LMWH (dalteparin, enoxaparin, tinzaparin, bemiparin) is the anticoagulant of choice, barring any special considerations (see below for special circumstances).

The dose is weight-related. Use the weight at booking or the current weight minus 10%.

> **!** To work out the dose required: dalteparin 100 units/kg SC twice daily, up to a maximum of 18 000 units.

Prescribe and use a prefilled syringe (from a choice of 2500, 5000, 10 000 and 12 500 units) nearest to the calculated requirement.

Do not use less than 10 000 units or more than 18 000 units in 24 hours.

Measure the peak anti-Xa level 3 hours post-injection, aiming for a therapeutic range of 0.5–1 units/mL. Adjust the level of dalteparin as advised by the haematologist, reassessing anti-Xa activity after each dose adjustment.

Check the platelet count on days 2 and 7 after commencement of dalteparin.

Intravenous unfractionated heparin

This has a shorter half-life than LMWH and is readily reversible with protamine sulphate, so should be considered in the following circumstances:

- massive PE
- floating thrombus on ultrasound scan
- prosthetic valve
- renal failure
- increased risk of bleeding (e.g. as result of coagulopathy, trauma, surgery or peptic ulcer)
- wound haematoma
- APH or PPH

Ensure that baseline clotting and platelet count are normal before starting.

- **Loading dose**: 5000 units IV over 5 minutes.
- **Maintenance infusion**: Use a preparation of 1000 units /mL. Start at 1 mL/h (i.e. 1000 units/h).

Check the APTT 4–6 hours after the loading dose, aiming for a therapeutic target of 2–2.5 times the average laboratory control value.

Adjust the infusion rate as advised by the haematologist, and recheck the APTT every 4–6 hours until the therapeutic ratio is reached. Once the therapeutic ratio is reached, check the APTT at least daily.

In some pregnancies, the therapeutic ratio is difficult to achieve despite high doses of heparin, because fibrinogen and factor VIII levels rise in pregnancy. In such cases, anti-Xa activity should be monitored, aiming for a range of 0.35–0.70 units /mL.

Check the platelet count on days 2, 7and 10.

Contraindications to heparin (including LMWH)

- active bleeding
- if surgical treatment is to be undertaken (e.g. a caval filter or an embolectomy)
- previous heparin-induced thrombocytopenia (use danaparoid)
- previous heparin skin allergy (discuss with the haematologist)

Duration of treatment

Following treatment of the acute phase, anticoagulation should be maintained with LMWH for at least 6 months. In many cases, it will be safe to reduce anticoagulation to a prophylactic dose. Arrange a follow-up appointment with the haematology/coagulation clinic.

Labour and delivery

A woman on therapeutic anticoagulation should be delivered by planned induction of labour or elective CS at 37–38 weeks. She should be advised that in the event of contractions starting before the day of admission, no further heparin should be self-administered until she has been assessed in hospital.

Women on a prophylactic dose may await spontaneous onset of labour.

Induction of labour

☐ Omit the evening dose of dalteparin before admission.
☐ On admission: FBC, coagulation profile, anti-Xa and group-and-save.
☐ Inform the haematologist.
☐ Dalteparin 5000 units daily (i.e. a prophylactic dose) should be given on admission and continued until the woman has delivered.
☐ Apply thromboembolism-deterrent stockings.
☐ There should be active management of the third stage.
☐ Give a Syntocinon (oxytocin) infusion 40 units in 500 mL Hartmann's solution or 0.9% saline for 4 hours post-delivery.
☐ The therapeutic regimen should be resumed following delivery.

Elective caesarean section

☐ Omit the evening dose of dalteparin before the day of operation.
☐ On admission: FBC, coagulation profile, anti-Xa and group-and-save.
☐ Inform the haematologist.
☐ Give dalteparin 5000 units SC 3 hours postoperative, or 4 hours after removal of the epidural catheter.
☐ Consider placing a wound drain.
☐ Use staples or interrupted sutures for skin.
☐ Give a Syntocinon infusion 40 units in 500 mL Hartmann's solution or 0.9% saline for 4 hours post-delivery.
☐ The therapeutic regimen should be resumed the evening after surgery.
☐ Apply thromboembolism-deterrent stockings.

Epidural or spinal anaesthesia

This should be discussed with the woman before induction of labour or CS.

- **If the woman is on a therapeutic dose of LMWH**, a regional block should not be used until at least 24 hours after the last dose.
- **If the woman is on a prophylactic dose** (this should be the case if the above protocol for induction and elective CS has been followed), a regional block should not be used until at least 12 hours after the last dose.

LMWH should not be given for at least 6 hours after the epidural catheter has been removed. The cannula should not be removed within 12 hours of the most recent injection.

Postpartum anticoagulation

Anticoagulation should be continued for at least 6 weeks. If the woman opts for an oral anticoagulant (warfarin), this can be started on the day following delivery. Breastfeeding is not a contraindication to warfarin.

60 Major haemoglobinopathy

The major haemoglobinopathies are sickle cell disease and thalassaemia. These should be excluded in women of African, Asian or Mediterranean origin. In particular, major haemoglobinopathy should be suspected when there is anaemia in the absence of bleeding in a woman from any of these populations (but haemoglobinopathy is not exclusive to them). A sickle cell crisis may be precipitated or exacerbated by hypoxia/acidosis, dehydration and infection.

Principles of management in labour

- Avoid dehydration, infection, acidosis, hypoxia and prolonged labour.
- Liaise with the haematologist and the blood transfusion laboratory.
- Inform the anaesthetist and paediatrician on admission.
- If administering a Syntocinon (oxytocin) drip, avoid fluid overload.
- In cases of PROM, labour should be induced to minimize the risk of chorioamnionitis.
- Do not give an iron supplement.

Action plan

☐ Record BP and do a urinalysis on admission.
☐ Check FBC, U/E, LFT, urates, creatinine and blood gases on admission.
☐ Establish IV access.
☐ Cross-match 4 units of blood.
☐ Initiate continuous CTG monitoring.
☐ Set up pulse oximetry.
☐ Administer oxygen.
☐ Provide a liberal oral fluid intake or judicious use of IV fluids.
☐ Give antibiotic cover – penicillin.
☐ Recommend epidural analgesia, especially where operative delivery is anticipated, but:
  - avoid overload when giving IV fluid before epidural
  - use elastic stockings and leg elevation to avoid hypotension and venous pooling in the legs.
☐ Watch for signs of PE.

☐   Consider thromboembolism prophylaxis.
☐   There should be active management of the third stage.
☐   Take cord blood for FBC and haemoglobin electrophoresis.

Sickle cell crisis

Bone pain crisis

- fever
- painful limbs, chest and abdomen
- tender bones and abdomen

Sequestration

- bone pain
- abdominal pain, fever
- hepatomegaly
- splenomegaly
- falling [Hb]

Aplastic crisis

- fever
- dyspnoea
- pallor
- low [Hb]
- low reticulocyte count

☐   Involve the haematologist.
☐   Maintain airway oxygen via a facemask, 15 L/min.
☐   Assess pulse and BP.
☐   Monitor O_2 saturation.
☐   ECG.
☐   Establish IV access: FBC, U/E, reticulocyte count and LFT.
☐   Check arterial blood gases.
☐   Do a sepsis screen: blood culture, and a midstream specimen of urine for bacteriology.
☐   Do a chest X-ray if there are chest symptoms.
☐   Rehydrate with Hartmann's solution or 0.9% saline.
☐   Monitor fluid input and urine output.
☐   Administer parenteral analgesia.
☐   Administer IV antibiotics.
☐   Treat the cause of the crisis if identified.

☐ Cross-match 4 units of blood (the laboratory must be informed that the woman has sickle cell disease).

☐ Give a transfusion as required (packed cells) – discuss with the haematologist. A transfusion is not usually required if [Hb] ≥ 6 g/dL.

61 Inherited coagulation disorders: haemophilia and von Willebrand disease

Coagulation disorders can be inherited or acquired:

- **Inherited**: haemophilia, von Willebrand disease, factor XI deficiency and other rare disorders.
- **Acquired**: gestational thrombocytopenia and immune thrombocytopenic purpura (ITP, Chapter 62).

Haemophilia

Haemophilia A is due to deficiency of factor VIII. Haemophilia B is due to deficiency of factor IX. Both are X-linked recessive disorders. Most carriers do not have bleeding problems, but a small number have a tendency to bleed, owing to low clotting factor levels that result from lyonization or homozygosity.

von Willebrand disease

This is a group of autosomally inherited disorders characterized by reduced synthesis of von Willebrand factor (vWF) or by structural or functional defects in this factor. vWF is essential for normal platelet function and acts as a carrier for factor VIII, so patients with von Willebrand disease usually have prolonged bleeding time and reduced factor VIIIc activity.

von Willebrand disease is classified into three types: in type 1, there is a partial deficiency in the production of vWF, but its structure and function are normal; in type 2 (of which there are a number of subtypes), the amount of vWF produced may be normal, but the structure and function are abnormal; in type 3, there is total or near total deficiency in vWF. Bleeding is more frequent and more severe in types 2 and 3. Type 1 is autosomal dominant, type 2 is usually autosomal dominant (rarely autosomal recessive) and type 3 is autosomal recessive.

The incidence of primary PPH is high, and the incidence of secondary PPH is even higher. In severe cases, discuss with the haematologist regarding treatment with desmopressin acetate (DDAVP) or vWF concentrate. Tranexamic acid 1 g three times daily should be given immediately following delivery and continued for 5 days. Secondary PPH may also be treated with tranexamic acid.

Action plan

- ☐ Check notes for the plan agreed with the consultant haematologist.
- ☐ Ascertain the availability of blood products as required (see below).
- ☐ FBC.
- ☐ Do coagulation tests.
- ☐ Check clotting factor levels (factor VIIIc in haemophilia A and factor IX in haemophilia B). If levels are <50 IU/dL, transfuse with recombinant factor VIII or IX and recheck 30 minutes after transfusion.
- ☐ Group-and-save.
- ☐ Avoid IM injections.
- ☐ Avoid NSAIDs.
- ☐ Epidural analgesia may be given, provided that the coagulation screen is normal and the platelet count is >100 × 10^9/L. Epidural analgesia is also considered safe if clotting factor levels are >50 IU/dL.
- ☐ Repeat the coagulation screen before removing the epidural catheter.
- ☐ Avoid the use of FSE and FBS, since an affected fetus may bleed (the sex of the unborn baby is not usually known).
- ☐ Make early recourse to CS in cases of slow progress.
- ☐ Avoid vacuum-assisted delivery (a low forceps delivery may be performed and is preferable to a traumatic CS delivery).
- ☐ If CS or instrumental delivery is required, ensure that clotting factor levels are >50 IU/L. If they are <50 IU/L, transfuse with recombinant factor VIII or IX, as appropriate.
- ☐ Anticipate PPH.
- ☐ Factor VIII and factor IX fall rapidly after delivery. Post-delivery, ensure that clotting factor activity is >50 IU/dL for 5 days, to minimize the risk of PPH.

The neonate

- ☐ Obtain cord blood in a citrated bottle from all male babies for investigation.
- ☐ Give the neonate oral vitamin K.
- ☐ Perform a cranial ultrasound scan if there is any suggestion of possible intracranial bleed (e.g. poor feeding, lethargy or vomiting).
- ☐ Inform the GP so that the neonate's immunizations are given subcutaneously or intradermally.

62 Immune thrombocytopenic purpura

Immune thrombocytopenic purpura (ITP) is a condition in which platelets are destroyed prematurely by antiplatelet antibodies. There is no diagnostic test – the condition is diagnosed by exclusion of other causes of thrombocytopenia. The platelet count is persistently low (<100 × 10^9/L), but the FBC, blood film, PT and APTT are normal. Tests for antiplatelet antibodies are non-specific and do not distinguish ITP from gestational thrombocytopenia. Bone marrow biopsy may be needed for diagnosis.

When seen on the delivery suite, the woman will fall into one of the following groups, depending on what treatment she has received:

- **Asymptomatic and with platelet count >50 × 10^9/L:** requires no treatment.
- **Been on prednisolone for maintenance of platelet count**: give hydrocortisone 100 mg IV every 8 hours to cover labour and delivery (because of inhibition of the pituitary–adrenal axis): watch for hyperglycaemia.
- **IV immunoglobulin given just before induction of labour or CS**: watch for side-effects of headache, nausea, alopecia and abnormal LFT.

Action plan

- ☐ Check notes for the plan agreed with the consultant haematologist.
- ☐ FBC.
- ☐ LFT.
- ☐ Obtain a coagulation profile.
- ☐ Check clotting factor levels.
- ☐ Confirm availability and access to platelets for transfusion.
- ☐ Alert paediatricians (the baby is at risk of thrombocytopenia, which carries a risk of intracranial haemorrhage).
- ☐ Avoid intramuscular injection of pethidine.
- ☐ Discuss pain relief with the consultant anaesthetist.
- ☐ Epidural is not contraindicated if:
  - FBC is normal
  - the coagulation profile is normal
  - clotting factor levels are >50 IU/L during the third trimester.

☐   Check factor levels before removing the epidural catheter.
☐   Obtain an anticoagulated cord blood sample and send it immediately to the haemophilia laboratory.

Mode of delivery

The mode of delivery in cases of ITP remains controversial. In each case, it should be decided by the consultant obstetrician and consultant haematologist, with the consent of the woman. If the platelet count is $<50 \times 10^9/L$ then platelet transfusion and CS may decrease the risk of intracranial haemorrhage in the neonate.

Avoid the use of FSE and vacuum-assisted delivery.

The neonate

Antiplatelet antibodies may cross the placenta, causing fetal thrombocytopenia. This may manifest as purpura, haematuria or intracranial haemorrhage. Neither prednisolone therapy nor IV immunoglobulin given to the mother can prevent fetal thrombocytopenia.

The risk of bleeding is low if the fetus has a platelet count of $>50 \times 10^9/L$, but obtaining a sample of fetal blood is risky and requires special skills.

Action

- Give vitamin K orally.
- Routine immunizations should be given subcutaneously or intradermally.
- Consider hepatitis B immunization.

63 Thrombophilia

Thrombophilia is an abnormality of haemostasis predisposing to thrombosis. It may be:

- **hereditary**:
  - activated protein C resistance (associated with factor V Leiden mutation)
  - protein C deficiency
  - protein S deficiency
  - antithrombin deficiency
  - prothrombin gene mutation
- **acquired**:
  - antiphospholipid syndrome
  - polycythaemia
  - other conditions (e.g. malignancy)

Hyperhomocysteinaemia is a thrombophilia with genetic and acquired origins.

About 50% of thromboembolic events in pregnancy occur in women with an identifiable thrombophilia.

Women with thrombophilia are also at increased risk of stillbirth, IUGR and pre-eclampsia.

Management in labour

Most women with known thrombophilia will have been commenced on anticoagulant treatment antenatally.

- ☐ Check the notes for the management plan as outlined by the consultant obstetrician or haematologist.
- ☐ Discontinue heparin/LMWH if in labour or before induction of labour.
- ☐ FBC.
- ☐ Do a coagulation screen: APTT, PT and anti-Xa assay (if available).
- ☐ Watch for pre-eclampsia developing in labour.

Epidural analgesia

This may be considered if:

- heparin/LMWH has not been given in the preceding 6 hours
- the coagulation screen is normal
- the platelet count is >100 × 10^9/L

Postpartum

- Resume anticoagulant prophylaxis 12 hours after delivery (unless bleeding is in excess of lochial loss).
- Continue anticoagulant prophylaxis for 3 months.
- Oral anticoagulants may be started within the first 2 days, and heparin/LMWH should be withdrawn when the International Normalized Ratio (INR) has been within the therapeutic range for 3 days.
- In cases of heritable thrombophilia, inform the parents of the risk of autosomal transmission.

64 Gestational thrombocytopenia

This is a mild reduction in platelet count occurring in the second or third trimester, with no bleeding problems for mother or baby. The platelet count is usually in the range $100–150 \times 10^9$/L and reverts to normal after pregnancy.

Vaginal delivery is safe.

Regional analgesia is safe.

Platelet count returns to normal 2–12 weeks after delivery.

65 Antepartum haemorrhage

Antepartum haemorrhage (APH) is defined formally as bleeding from the genital tract after 24 weeks' gestation. In practice, vaginal bleeding that occurs after a woman has had a normal fetal anatomy scan is managed as APH.

Differential diagnosis

- placenta praevia (Chapter 66)
- placental abruption (concealed bleeding could be more significant than revealed loss)
- bleeding from the cervix (ectopy, polyp, carcinoma, etc.)
- vasa praevia

Assessment

- ☐ Assess blood loss.
- ☐ Check BP, pulse and respiration.
- ☐ If the woman is in shock: airway, breathing, circulation.
- ☐ Exclude abdominal pain and contractions.
- ☐ Exclude placenta praevia before performing a digital vaginal examination.

> **!** Note that abruption of a posterior placenta may present as back pain.

Minor APH (minimal loss on admission)

- ☐ Check scan reports for placental site (but note that scans can be wrong).
- ☐ Perform a speculum examination.
- ☐ FBC, group-and-save; do a Kleihauer test if the woman is Rh-negative.
- ☐ CTG.
- ☐ If the woman is Rh-negative, give anti-D 1000 units IM.
- ☐ Transfer to the ward if there is no major bleeding, uterine tenderness or fetal distress.

Moderate APH (significant bleeding but not in shock)

☐ Insert an IV line (14G). Crystalloid infusion.

☐ FBC, U/E, clotting, cross-match 4 units; do a Kleihauer test if the woman is Rh-negative.

☐ Catheterize and monitor urine output.

☐ Set up an intensive monitoring chart.

☐ Inform the anaesthetist and neonatal unit.

☐ Inform the consultant: a decision must be made regarding the mode and timing of delivery.

☐ If the woman is Rh-negative and delivery is not imminent, give anti-D 1000 units IM.

☐ Monitor on the delivery suite for up to 12 hours post-delivery.

Major APH (estimated loss > 1000 mL)

☐ Call for a senior obstetrician, anaesthetist, theatre team and porters. Alert the blood bank and haematology laboratory.

☐ Administer oxygen by mask: 8 L/min.

☐ Keep the woman warm.

☐ Insert two IV lines with 14G, or larger, cannulae.

☐ Catheterize and monitor urine output.

☐ ECG.

☐ Set up pulse oximetry.

☐ Initiate serial BP recording.

☐ Consider CVP monitoring and an arterial line. This is likely to be required if blood loss is in excess of 1500 mL or if the woman is to be taken to theatre.

> **!** 'Failure to use [CVP] monitoring in the treatment of major obstetric haemorrhage is substandard care.'
>
> Thomas TA, Cooper GM. Anaesthesia. In: Lewis G, ed. *Why Mothers Die 1997–1999. The Confidential Enquiries into Maternal Deaths in the United Kingdom.* London: RCOG Press, 2001: 143

☐ FBC, PT, APTT, FDP and fibrinogen.

☐ Urgently cross-match 6 units of blood.

☐ Give plasma substitutes: Haemaccel or Gelofusine 1000 mL immediately.

☐ Transfuse cross-matched blood if available.

☐ If cross-matched blood is not available immediately, use:
  • unmatched blood (patient's group), which is usually available within 15 minutes
  • group O negative blood (emergency stock) – if blood is needed immediately.

☐ **Before using uncross-matched blood, always:**
  • **discuss with the laboratory**
  • **obtain the woman's blood sample for tests listed above.**

☐ Use 1 unit FFP for every 8 units of packed cells. Further transfusion of coagulation factors may be required – see 'Transfusion of clotting factors' below.

> **!** Blood-warming equipment should be used.

☐ Continuous CTG monitoring.

☐ Record blood loss: weigh soaked linen.

☐ If CTG is normal and bleeding has settled, perform an ultrasound scan. A scan is also indicated if fetal heart tones are not detected.

Transfusion of clotting factors

The clinical situation may have changed by the time blood results are available, so treat the patient not the results. Treat coagulation defects as advised by the haematologist. Transfusion of FFP is usually required if blood loss/replacement approaches the estimated blood volume of the woman. Platelet transfusion is usually needed with 1.5–2 times blood volume replacement. Cryoprecipitate is likely to be needed if the fibrinogen level is abnormally low.

> 'A standing agreement between the haematologists and obstetricians over the issue of platelets, FFP and cryoprecipitate reduces the number of phone calls required and speeds response. Coagulation monitoring will help to assess the adequacy of the coagulation support and guide the selection of components but should not delay the initial issue of FFP or cryoprecipitate.'
>
> Blood Transfusion Services of the United Kingdom. Obstetric haemorrhage. In: McClelland DBL, ed. *Handbook of Transfusion Medicine*, 3rd edn. London: The Stationery Office, 2001: 80

The senior obstetrician makes the decision regarding urgency and mode of delivery.

Consider early transfer to ITU/HDU.

Delivery

There should be active management of the third stage of labour.

APH predisposes to PPH, so a Syntocinon (oxytocin) infusion (40 units in 500 mL Hartmann's solution or 0.9% saline) should be commenced in the third stage of labour and continued for 4 hours post-delivery.

66 Major placenta praevia

Vaginal delivery is contraindicated if the placenta encroaches within 2 cm of the internal os.

Elective or emergency CS for major placenta praevia should be performed only by a consultant obstetrician or by an experienced obstetrician with the consultant in attendance.

Action plan

☐ Discuss the possibility of blood transfusion.

☐ Cross-match 4–6 units of blood.

☐ Liaise with interventional radiologist.

☐ In cases of anterior placenta praevia in a scarred uterus (i.e. previous CS), the woman should be informed of the possibility of placenta accreta.

☐ Consent should be obtained for a hysterectomy to be performed in the event of uncontrollable bleeding.

☐ Anticipate PPH: commence Syntocinon (oxytocin) infusion (40 units in 500 mL Hartmann's solution or 0.9% saline) immediately after delivery of the baby.

> **!** In the event of massive haemorrhage, manage as outlined on pp. 191–2.

67 Retained placenta

By definition, 'retained placenta' occurs when the placenta has shown no signs of separation after 20 minutes of delivery of the baby (60 minutes if the third stage has been managed physiologically).

The plan below also applies when the placenta has been delivered but there are missing cotyledons.

> **!** In the case of a scarred uterus, beware of placenta accreta. Obtain consent for possible blood transfusion and hysterectomy before proceeding to manual removal.

In some cases of retained placenta, the placenta will separate following injection of a mixture of Syntocinon (oxytocin) 10–20 units and 20 mL 0.9% saline into the umbilical vein.

Action plan

- ☐ Inform the registrar.
- ☐ Ensure that the bladder is empty.
- ☐ Insert an IV line (14G or larger).
- ☐ Give a Syntocinon infusion 40 units in 500 mL Hartmann's solution or 0.9% saline.
- ☐ Group-and-save (cross-match if bleeding is >500 mL).
- ☐ Monitor pulse, BP and blood loss.
- ☐ Counsel the woman regarding the possibility of placenta accreta.
- ☐ Remove the retained placenta manually in theatre under spinal or epidural analgesia. (A general anaesthetic is preferable only if the patient is shocked or bleeding heavily.)
- ☐ If the placenta is morbidly adherent, call the consultant immediately.
- ☐ Continue Syntocinon infusion for 4 hours after manual removal.
- ☐ Give IV co-amoxiclav (Augmentin) or cefuroxime/metronidazole as a bolus.
- ☐ If uterine inversion occurs during the process of manual removal then reduce the inversion before any further attempt at removing the placenta. Call the consultant immediately. See also Chapter 83.

68 Postpartum haemorrhage

> **!** Only two-thirds of all postpartum haemorrhages (PPH) occur in women with known risk factors.

> **!** At CS, blood loss is likely to be higher if the placenta is removed manually than if it were removed by cord traction.

Action plan

- ☐ Summon help.
- ☐ For major haemorrhage:
  - Call the team leader, obstetricians, anaesthetist, porter and other members of the theatre team.
  - Alert the blood bank and haematologist.
  - Nominate a recorder.
- ☐ Assess airway, breathing and circulation.
- ☐ Give uterine massage.
- ☐ Administer oxygen by mask.
- ☐ Keep the woman warm.
- ☐ Catheterize and monitor urine output.
- ☐ Assess blood loss.
- ☐ Insert two wide-bore IV cannulae (14G or larger).
- ☐ FBC and clotting profile.
- ☐ Urgent cross-match 6 units.
- ☐ Give oxytocic drugs, as may be required, in the following order:
  - Syntocinon (oxytocin) 10 units IM bolus
  - Syntocinon infusion 40 units in 500 mL Hartmann's solution
  - ergometrine 0.5 mg IV (an antiemetic may be given simultaneously)
  - carboprost (Hemabate) 0.25 mg IM, repeated every 15 minutes, up to eight doses (maximum dose 2 mg).
- ☐ Give plasma substitutes: IV Haemaccel or Gelofusine 1.5 L immediately.
- ☐ Institute serial BP monitoring.
- ☐ Consider CVP monitoring.

> **!** 'Failure to use [CVP] monitoring in the treatment of major obstetric haemorrhage is substandard care.'
>
> Thomas TA, Cooper GM. Anaesthesia. In: Lewis G, ed. *Why Mothers Die 1997–1999. The Confidential Enquiries into Maternal Deaths in the United Kingdom.* London: RCOG Press, 2001: 143

- ☐ Record pulse rate, BP, O$_2$ saturation, CVP and other observations on a high-dependency chart.
- ☐ Diagnose and treat the source of bleeding – 'the four Ts':
  Tone
  Trauma
  Tissue (placenta)
  Thrombin (clotting)

Retained placenta

Proceed immediately to manual removal.

Uterine atony

Give an oxytocic regimen as above. Also consider the use of a Bakri or Sengstaken–Blakemore tube. Before using the tube, ensure that there are no retained products of conception. Inflate the balloon with sterile fluid (see product label for maximum volume). Leave for 24 hours, and then deflate. The Bakri balloon has an inner lumen which enables assessment of ongoing blood loss.

Genital tract trauma or undiagnosed bleeding

Proceed to EUA. Counsel for laparotomy and possible hysterectomy. Good light and good assistance are essential for EUA.

Coagulopathy

Manage in collaboration with a haematologist. The clinical situation may have changed by the time blood results are available, so treat the patient not the results. Treat coagulation defects as advised by the haematologist. Transfusion of FFP is usually required if blood loss/replacement approaches the estimated blood volume of the woman. Platelet transfusion is usually needed with 1.5–2 times blood volume replacement. Cryoprecipitate is likely to be needed if the fibrinogen level is abnormally low.

> 'A standing agreement between the haematologists and obstetricians over the issue of platelets, FFP and cryoprecipitate reduces the number of phone calls required and speeds response. Coagulation monitoring will help to assess the adequacy of the coagulation support and guide the selection of components but should not delay the initial issue of FFP or cryoprecipitate.'
>
> Blood Transfusion Services of the United Kingdom. Obstetric haemorrhage. In: McClelland DBL, ed. *Handbook of Transfusion Medicine*, 3rd edn. London: The Stationery Office, 2001: 80

- [ ] The frequency of repeat blood tests is determined by the clinical situation, but in major bleeding this is usually every 4 hours until stable.
- [ ] Estimate the blood loss: weigh soaked linen and swabs.
- [ ] Consider early transfer to HDU or ITU.

> **!** **Take care**: in the rush to get things done, a blood specimen is sometimes sent to the laboratory either unlabelled or with incorrect identity.

Blood transfusion

- [ ] Transfuse cross-matched blood if available.
- [ ] If cross-matched blood is not available immediately, use:
  - unmatched blood (patient's group), which is usually available within 15 minutes
  - group O negative blood (emergency stock) – if blood is needed immediately (i.e. in a life-threatening situation).
- [ ] **Before using uncross-matched blood, always**:
  - **discuss with the laboratory**
  - **obtain the woman's blood sample for the tests listed above.**
- [ ] Use blood-warming equipment.
- [ ] Infuse with a pressure bag.

Where do things usually go wrong?

- Failure to anticipate high-risk patients.
- Being falsely reassured by a systolic BP > 100 mmHg. Usually systolic pressure does not fall until a minimum of 1.5 L has been lost.
- Inadequate blood transfusion or excessive use of fluids.
- Failure to detect early DIC and respond appropriately.
- Lack of involvement of senior staff at an early stage.
- Delay in resort to surgical treatment.

Documentation:
The nature, time and outcome of any intervention should be documented (free text or proforma).

69 Disseminated intravascular coagulopathy

Disseminated intravascular coagulopathy (DIC) should be anticipated in severe pre-eclampsia, APH, PPH, placental abruption, amniotic fluid embolism and septicaemia.

Early involvement of the haematologist is vital.

Investigations

- ☐ FBC.
- ☐ Group and cross-match 4–6 units of blood.
- ☐ Obtain a coagulation profile.

Low fibrinogen and elevated FDP levels are indicative of decompensation. Serial measurements of haemastatic indices are more informative than single readings.

Treatment

- High-dependency care is necessary.
- Manage shock.
- Liaise with the consultant haematologist (regarding blood product support).
- Treat the underlying cause – this is the cornerstone of management.
- See the protocol for management of massive haemorrhage (pp. 191–2).

70 Delivery of the woman at known risk of haemorrhage

A higher risk of major bleeding at delivery should be anticipated in the following cases:

- previous PPH
- placenta praevia
- significant uterine fibroids
- previous myomectomy
- placental abruption
- multiple pregnancy
- APH
- significant uterine fibroids
- grandmultiparity
- retained placenta
- macrosomia
- prolonged labour

Women at risk should have:

- a 14FG IV cannula during labour
- FBC and group-and-save on admission
- their bladder emptied in the third stage of labour
- active management of the third stage of labour

A Syntocinon (oxytocin) infusion 40 units in 50 mL 0.9% saline (or Hartmann's) should be given for 4 hours after delivery.

When surgery is indicated

All elective and emergency surgery should be performed by a consultant or by an experienced obstetrician, with a consultant in attendance.

A senior anaesthetist should be involved. Elective CS for placenta praevia and other potentially difficult cases should be scheduled for a session when a consultant anaesthetist is available.

☐   Place two 14FG IV cannulae before surgery.

☐ Cross-match 4 units of blood. These should be immediately available.

☐ Insert a CVP line (either preoperatively or when bleeding is excessive).

Liaise with the consultant haematologist in cases of coagulopathy.

See also management of PPH (Chapter 68) and management of major placenta praevia (Chapter 66).

71 Management of the woman who declines blood transfusion

Some women decline transfusion because of specific personal or religious beliefs. The main group of women who may refuse for religious reasons are members of the Jehovah's Witnesses.

If it is thought likely that a woman may refuse blood transfusion then management of massive haemorrhage should be considered in advance.

Antenatal care

Discuss the risks of withholding blood transfusion (in a non-confrontational, non-judgemental manner). The woman should be offered the opportunity to read and discuss the guidance given below.

She should be asked if she is willing to receive blood transfusion in a life-threatening emergency, and her reply should be noted. This reply, given without duress, constitutes an advance decision. She should sign the appropriate form indicating her refusal of blood or blood products.

A copy of her Advance Decision document should be in her hospital records. It should be clear what interventions she will accept and which ones she does not want:

- ☐ whole blood
- ☐ red cells
- ☐ white cells
- ☐ platelets
- ☐ FFP
- ☐ blood products:
  - ☐ albumin
  - ☐ cryoprecipitate
  - ☐ immunoglobulin
  - ☐ coagulation factors
- ☐ autologous transfusion using blood salvage systems

Check blood group and antibody status at booking, 30 weeks and 36 weeks.

Arrange a consultation with the consultant obstetric anaesthetist.

Check haemoglobin and serum ferritin at 36 weeks.

Haematinics should be given throughout pregnancy to maximize iron stores.

If an ultrasound scan shows a low-lying placenta then the implications should be discussed with the woman.

> **!** Blood storage for autotransfusion should not be suggested to pregnant women, since the amounts of blood required to treat massive obstetric haemorrhage are far in excess of the amount that could be donated during pregnancy.

The consultant obstetrician must be kept informed of any antenatal complications.

Labour

- [ ] On admission, inform the consultant obstetrician and consultant anaesthetist.
- [ ] Review the antenatal assessment as outlined above.
- [ ] Confirm with the woman what her wishes are.
- [ ] Note whether she is taking any drugs that could cause or aggravate bleeding.
- [ ] If a blood salvage device is to be used, alert the perfusionist.
- [ ] The third stage of labour should be managed actively.
- [ ] The woman should be observed closely for at least an hour after delivery.

If CS is necessary, it should be carried out by a consultant obstetrician if possible.

When the mother is discharged from hospital, she should be advised to report any bleeding promptly.

Management of haemorrhage

The principle is to avoid delay. Rapid decision-making may be necessary, particularly with regard to surgical intervention.

- [ ] Inform the consultant obstetrician.
- [ ] Inform the consultant anaesthetist.

☐   Inform the consultant haematologist.

☐   Promptly commence standard management (short of blood transfusion) of APH and PPH (Chapters 65 and 68).

The threshold for intervention should be lower than in other patients.

Extra vigilance should be exercised to quantify any abnormal bleeding and to detect complications, such as clotting abnormalities, as promptly as possible.

Communication

- Keep the woman fully informed about what is happening. Information must be given in a professional way, ideally by someone whom the woman knows and trusts.
- Maintain a professional attitude. Do not lose the trust of the patient or her partner, since further decisions (e.g. regarding hysterectomy) may have to be made.
- If standard treatment is not controlling the bleeding, advise the woman that blood transfusion is strongly recommended. She is entitled to change her mind about a previously agreed treatment plan.
- Be satisfied that the woman is not being subjected to pressure from others. It is reasonable to ask the accompanying persons to leave the room for a while so that the doctor (with a midwife or other colleague) can ask the woman whether she is making her decision of her own free will.
- If the woman maintains her refusal to accept blood or blood products then her wishes must be respected.

Drugs and infusions

Dextran should be avoided for fluid replacement because of its possible effects on haemostasis. IV crystalloid and plasma substitutes (Haemaccel or Gelofusine) should be used. In cases of severe bleeding, IV vitamin K should be given to the woman. Other drugs that have been recommended include desmopressin, methylprednisolone and inhibitors of fibrinolysis, such as aprotinin and tranexamic acid.

The advice of the haematologist should be sought before considering the use of heparin to combat DIC.

If the woman survives the acute episode and is transferred to ITU, management there should include erythropoietin, parenteral iron therapy and adequate protein for haemoglobin synthesis.

Hysterectomy

Hysterectomy is usually a treatment of last resort in obstetric haemorrhage, but for a woman who declines blood transfusion any delay may increase the risk of death. The timing of hysterectomy is an on-the-spot decision for the consultant.

When hysterectomy is performed, the uterine arteries should be clamped as early as possible in the procedure. Subtotal hysterectomy can be just as effective as total hysterectomy, and is quicker and safer.

In some cases, there may be a place for ligation of the internal iliac artery.

> **!** If, in spite of all care, the woman dies then her relatives require support like any other bereaved family.

Management of staff

It is distressing for staff to have to watch a woman bleed to death while refusing effective treatment. Support should be available for staff in these circumstances.

SECTION 4
Infection

72 Prophylactic antibiotics

Caesarean section

All women undergoing elective or emergency CS should have a single-dose prophylactic antibiotic: IV cefuroxime 750 mg given after clamping of the cord.

If there are two or more of the following risk factors for postoperative wound infection then consider giving a full course of antibiotics:

- prolonged rupture of membranes (>12 hours)
- prolonged labour (>8 hours)
- multiple vaginal examinations (>5 in the past 24 hours)
- obesity (body mass index > 30 kg/m² at booking)

Cardiac disease

All women in labour and with a structural heart defect, prosthetic valve or history of endocarditis must have prophylactic antibiotics:

- **CS**: amoxicillin 1 g IV and gentamicin 120 mg IV (over 3 minutes) at induction of anaesthesia, then amoxicillin 500 mg 6 hours later.
- **Vaginal delivery**: amoxicillin 1 g IV and gentamicin 120 mg IV (over 3 minutes) at onset of labour or ruptured membranes, then amoxicillin 500 mg 6 hours later.
- **Woman allergic to penicillin or who has had more than a single dose of penicillin in the previous month**: vancomycin 1 g by slow IV infusion (over at least 60 minutes) before delivery, then gentamicin 120 mg IV at induction of anaesthesia or at rupture of membranes.

Group B streptococci (GBS)

See Chapter 75.

Prolonged rupture of fetal membranes

Commence prophylactic antibiotics after 18 hours. Follow the same regimen as for GBS (Chapter 75). See also antibiotic use in PROM (p. 24).

73 Intrapartum pyrexia

Inadequate treatment of intraoperative pyrexia can lead to escalation of sepsis and substantial maternal morbidity.

Principles

- Look for a focus of infection: respiratory, cardiac, urinary tract or other.
- Treat empirically with antibiotics while awaiting test results. Seek the advice of a microbiologist at an early stage regarding appropriate antibiotic therapy.
- The most common organism responsible for life-threatening infection in pregnant women is the beta-haemolytic *Streptococcus pyogenes* (Lancefield Group A); the most appropriate antibiotic for this is a combination of Tazocin (piperacillin and the beta-lactamase inhibitor tazobactam) and an aminoglycoside.
- Beware of VTE presenting as pyrexia.
- Watch for fetal tachycardia.

Action plan

☐ FBC
☐ U/E
☐ CRP
☐ CTG
☐ Send a specimen for culture:
  - vaginal swab
  - endocervical swab
  - midstream urine
  - blood
  - sputum and/or throat swab, if respiratory symptoms present
☐ IV antibiotics: co-amoxiclav 1.2 g every 8 hours or cefuroxime 1.5 g + metronidazole 500 mg every 8 hours will suffice as first-line therapy in women who are pyrexial but otherwise well
☐ In severe cases, add gentamicin or consider Tazocin (discuss with the microbiologist)
☐ Inform the paediatrician
☐ Record temperature hourly
☐ Watch for deterioration to severe sepsis or septic shock.
☐ Post-delivery, send the following for culture:
  - swabs from baby
  - placental swab

74 Hepatitis B and C

In the case of a woman infected with hepatitis B or C virus (HBV or HCV), the aim is to reduce the chances of transmitting infection to the baby and/or staff. The risk of neonatal infection is variable.

Elective CS is not routinely indicated for HBV or HCV, but may be offered to women co-infected with HCV and HIV

Mother-to-child transmission of HBV can be reduced by giving the baby passive (immunoglobulin) and active (vaccination) immunization.

Action plan

☐ Admit into a designated room.
☐ Check the case notes for any instructions from the virologist regarding management.
☐ Universal precautions apply – wear disposable apron, gown, gloves, mask and spectacles.
☐ For CS and repair of episiotomy/perineal tear, consider the use of blunt needles.
☐ Obtain cord blood for hepatitis B surface antigen (HBsAg) and e core antibody (HBeAb).
☐ Disinfect boots, bed and other material with antiseptic.
☐ Immunize the baby and confirm that an immunization schedule is in place.

> **!** • Do not use an FSE.
> • Do not perform FBS.

Immunization

Hepatitis B immunoglobulin: 200 IU IM, single dose, given within 24 hours of birth.

Hepatitis B vaccine: 10 mg IM, within 24 hours of birth and at 1, 2 and 12 months.

Breastfeeding

It is safe for a mother with Hepatitis B or Hepatitis C to breastfeed her baby immediately after birth. As there is no vaccination against Hepatitis C for the baby, breastfeeding should be temporarily stopped if the women's nipples or areola is cracked or bleeding.

75 Intrapartum antibiotic prophylaxis for group B streptococci

Principles

From 1% to 2% of babies born to women who carry group B streptococci (GBS) will develop clinical infection. Although this transmission rate is low, the fatality rate in affected babies is high (15–50%). Premature infants have a 10–15 times greater risk of acquiring GBS than do full-term infants.

Intrapartum antibiotic prophylaxis prevents vertical transmission and early-onset neonatal GBS.

Risk factors

- labour at <35 weeks' gestation
- prolonged rupture of membranes (>18 hours)
- intrapartum pyrexia (>38°C, 100.4°F) – see p. 208.
- previous delivery of an infant with GBS
- GBS urinary tract infection
- previous HVS showing GBS
- previous baby with neonatal GBS infection

Action plan

For all women falling in the at-risk groups listed above:

☐ Send a low vaginal swab for culture.

☐ Check for allergy to penicillin.

☐ Give benzylpenicillin (penicillin G) 3 g IV load as soon as possible after onset of labour, then give 1.5 g every 4 hours until delivery. **If the woman is allergic to penicillin, give clindamycin 900 mg IV every 8 hours until she has delivered**.

☐ If GBS is confirmed, flag the notes (a GBS sticker is available for this purpose).

☐ If GBS is confirmed, ensure that the woman is informed fully. Emphasize the need for prophylactic antibiotics.

Intrapartum antibiotic prophylaxis is not required for women undergoing CS in the absence of labour and with intact membranes.

The baby should be managed as outlined in Figure 75.1.

Useful contact for patients

Group B Strep Support
  PO Box 203
  Haywards Heath
  West Sussex
  RH16 1GF

  Tel: 01444 416176
  www.gbss.org.uk

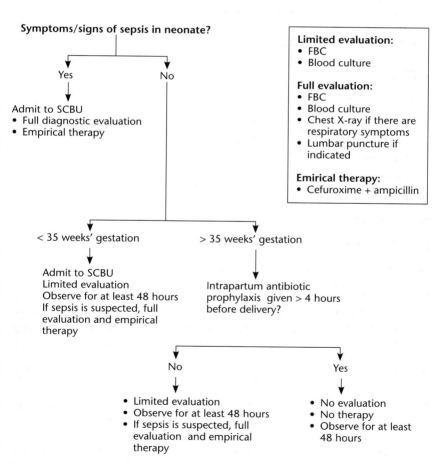

Figure 75.1 Management of a neonate whose mother received intrapartum antibiotic prophylaxis for GBS.

76 Genital herpes

About 90% of cases of genital herpes are caused by herpes simplex virus (HSV) type 2. It may present as painful vesicles or shallow ulcers, but there may be asymptomatic cervical lesions.

It may be a new (primary) infection or a recurrence. The risk of transmission to the baby is higher with primary infection (about 40%) than with recurrent infection (about 3%).

If a primary infection is present at term or in labour then elective CS should be offered; this reduces the risk of transmitting the infection to the baby.

Woman with a vesicular lesion or a history of genital herpes

☐ Examine the vulva and cervix.
☐ Obtain a cervical swab (and a vulval swab if lesions present) for viral culture if the diagnosis in doubt.
☐ If active herpes is present and fetal membranes are intact (or have just ruptured), offer CS:
  • For primary (first-episode) infection, this is the recommended mode of delivery.
  • For recurrent infection, the risk to the baby is small and must be weighed against the risk to the mother of a CS.
☐ If more than 4 hours have elapsed since membranes ruptured, ascending infection is likely to have occurred and CS is unlikely to reduce the risk of neonatal infection.
☐ Alert the paediatricians.
☐ Consult the genito-urinary physicians.
☐ Avoid invasive procedures such as amniotomy, FSE and FBS.
☐ Note that the use of aciclovir in pregnancy is off-label.

! It may be difficult to distinguish clinically between primary and recurrent genital herpes. If in doubt, treat as primary.

The decision pathway shown in Figure 76.1 is recommended.

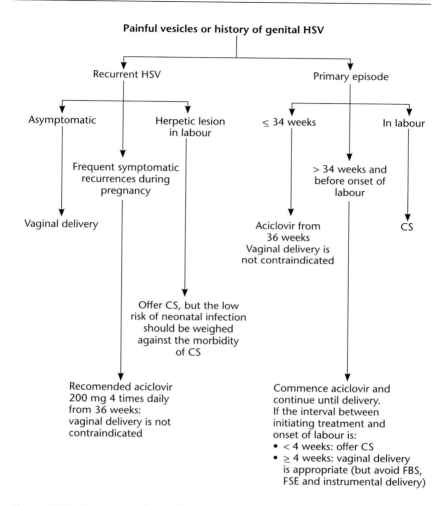

Figure 76.1 Decision pathway for mode of delivery in a woman with genital herpes.

77 Human immunodeficiency virus

The following events increase the risk of vertical transmission of Human immunodeficiency virus (HIV):

- vaginal delivery
- rupture of membranes >4 hours before delivery
- preterm delivery (particularly <34 weeks)
- use of FSE
- FBS
- chorioamnionitis
- breastfeeding
- high maternal viral load

In women who have been treated appropriately with antiretroviral drugs, <10% of babies become infected with HIV.

Elective CS (usually at 38 weeks) with intact membranes reduces the risk of vertical transmission by at least 50%. However, if the mother has been on antiretroviral therapy and viral load is undetectable then vaginal delivery will carry about the same risk of vertical transmission as elective CS.

Regional analgesia is not contraindicated.

Management of vaginal delivery

☐ Alert the paediatrician.

☐ Treat any intercurrent infection.

☐ If the woman is on antiretroviral therapy, continue until delivery.

☐ Start zidovudine when in established labour or rupture of membranes is confirmed. The initial dose is 2 mg/kg IV over 1 hour (use the woman's weight at booking), and this is followed by 1 mg/kg/h until the cord is clamped. To prepare the required dilution:

- Remove 100 mL from a 500 mL bag of 5% glucose, leaving 400 mL.
- Take five vials each containing 20 mL of zidovudine at 10 mg/mL, and add this to the 400 mL of 5% glucose. This gives a solution of 1000 mg zidovudine in 500 mL, i.e. a concentration of 2 mg/mL. This may be kept for 24 hours if necessary.
- With this concentration, if the woman's weight is x (kg) then the *loading infusion rate* will be x (mL/h) and the *maintenance infusion rate* will be $0.5x$ (mL/h).

☐ If the woman is not on (or has only recently started) zidovudine, recommend nevirapine 200 mg orally immediately at onset of labour, and start IV zidovudine (see the regime above).

☐ Cleanse the vagina with chlorhexidine. Use Hibitane cream instead of KY Jelly.

☐ Avoid ARM, if possible.

☐ Expedite delivery if there is inadequate uterine activity after spontaneous rupture of membranes.

☐ The active phase of the second stage of labour should not exceed 1 hour.

Other measures to reduce the risk of vertical transmission

- The use of FSE and FBS is absolutely contraindicated.
- Avoid episiotomy, if possible.
- If instrumental delivery is required, use forceps rather than ventouse.
- Clamp the cord as quickly as possible after delivery.
- Suction the baby's mouth (**not trachea**) and nose immediately after delivery.
- Wash the baby immediately after birth in a warm bath.
- Recommend formula feeding. However, if the mother opts to breastfeed then respect her decision and support her.
- Administer antiretroviral medication to the baby as prescribed (liaise with the paediatricians).

After delivery

- Arrange a follow-up appointment in clinic.
- Maintain confidentiality.

Preparation for caesarean section

- Start zidovudine infusion 4 hours before operation. The initial dose is 2 mg/kg IV over 1 hour, followed by 1 mg/kg/h until the cord is clamped.
- Universal infection control measures apply.
- Use blunt needles.
- Use staples for skin.

Prelabour rupture of membranes
Preterm

Assessment will have to be made as to the risk of HIV transmission compared with the risk of premature delivery. This assessment should involve obstetric, paediatric and infectious diseases staff. There is no known contraindication to the use of short-term steroids to promote fetal lung maturity in women with HIV.

At term

Manage actively, aiming to keep the interval between rupture of membranes and delivery less than 4 hours.

Cord blood

Cord blood should be taken for ultrasensitive HIV polymerase chain reaction (PCR), preferably in two EDTA bottles (one EDTA bottle will suffice if a sample sufficient to fill two bottles cannot be obtained). A clinical virology form must be completed, and 'ultrasensitive HIV PCR' must be written on the form.

To minimize needlestick injuries, a segment of cord should be steadied using two pairs of forceps.

Care of the baby

- Skin-to-skin contact should be established as soon as possible, unless declined by the mother.
- Bathe the baby.
- Administer vitamin K promptly, unless consent has been withheld.
- Administer antiretroviral therapy: nevirapine 2 mg/kg orally, one dose only, within 72 hours of birth (the sooner the better), and zidovudine 2 mg/kg every 6 hours orally, starting within 6 hours of birth and continued for 6 weeks.
- If the baby is premature or unable to tolerate oral medication, liaise with the HIV physician for IV medication.

Infection control

- Any needlestick injury should be managed as stipulated in the hospital policy.
- Standard personal protection equipment should be worn when undertaking any invasive procedures.

> **!** Attach a 'Biohazard' label to blood specimens.

SECTION 5
Other obstetric emergencies

78 Cervical tear and paravaginal haematoma

Paravaginal haematoma may manifest as shock, in the absence of significant bleeding.

- Examine in theatre under general anaesthesia or epidural analgesia.
- At examination under anaesthesia, ensure adequate exposure, with good lighting and an assistant.
- Assess whether blood transfusion is required (there is a tendency to underestimate blood loss).

Cervical tear

- Examine the cervix clockwise by serial clamping with sponge-holding forceps.
- The apex of the tear must be identified. If the apex cannot be seen then a laparotomy is indicated.

Paravaginal haematoma

- Ensure complete evacuation of the haematoma. A large incision may be required.
- After evacuation and repair, a tight pack should be inserted in the vagina.
- Give IV antibiotic: co-amoxiclav or cefuroxime/metronidazole.

79 Rupture of the uterus

Early diagnosis depends on a high index of suspicion.
Suspect a ruptured uterus if there is:

- sudden sharp abdominal pain followed by cessation of uterine contractions
- abdominal tenderness
- fetal distress (usually bradycardia)
- vaginal bleeding
- maternal collapse
- haematuria

> **!** Any of the above in the presence of a uterine scar is strongly suggestive of uterine rupture.

Action plan

- ☐ Call the senior obstetrician and anaesthetist.
- ☐ Maintain the airway with oxygen via a facemask.
- ☐ Assess pulse and BP.
- ☐ Obtain IV access (14G or larger).
- ☐ FBC and clotting screen, and cross-match 6 units.
- ☐ Give IV Hartmann's solution and blood transfusion as necessary.
- ☐ Give CPR if necessary.
- ☐ Set up continuous CTG (apply a scalp electrode).
- ☐ Obtain consent for laparotomy, and possible hysterectomy, under general anaesthetic. The extent of the operation will depend on the extent of rupture, the amount of bleeding and the patient's future reproductive intentions.
- ☐ Give IV co-amoxiclav or cefuroxime/metronidazole.

Preventive care

In contemporary practice, most women who suffer a ruptured uterus have had a previous CS or an oxytocic drug, or both. All women undergoing a trial of vaginal delivery after CS should be informed of the risk of scar rupture (approximately 1%).

In the presence of a uterine scar, a prostaglandin or Syntocinon (oxytocin) infusion should be used only with the prior approval of a consultant obstetrician, and the woman must be informed of the threefold increase in the risk of scar rupture.

Induction of labour in women with a previous CS should be in accordance with the protocol shown in Figure 34.3.

Vaginal birth after a previous CS should be managed as outlined in Chapter 33.

With Syntocinon induction or augmentation of labour, there should be continuous electronic fetal monitoring, and as much attention should be paid to the tocograph as to the cardiograph.

80 Shoulder dystocia

Risk factors

- large baby
- diabetes
- previous shoulder dystocia
- secondary arrest after 8 cm cervical dilatation
- instrumental delivery

> **!**
> - 50% of shoulder dystocia occurs in normal-sized babies.
> - More than 90% of macrosomic babies do not have dystocia.

Risks to mother and baby

- birth asphyxia
- fractures
- brachial plexus damage
- perineal trauma

When shoulder dystocia is anticipated

- Discuss with the woman.
- Give epidural analgesia early in labour.
- Deliver in the lithotomy position.
- The registrar should be present at delivery.

Turtle sign

The key to avoiding obstetric brachial plexus injury is to recognize, and respond appropriately to, the turtle sign. This is when the baby's head retracts against the mother's perineum (as a result of the baby's anterior shoulder impacting against the maternal pubic bone) – similar to a turtle pulling its head back into its shell. The baby's cheeks bulge out, its chin presses tightly on the perineum (you may find that you have to push back the perineum in order to deliver the chin), and the neck is not seen.

Once this sign appears, there should be no traction on the baby's head until the action plan below has been

executed. When traction is subsequently applied, it should be axial, with no lateral flexion of the neck.

Action plan: 'HELPERR'

- ☐ **Help**: Call for help: senior obstetrician, second midwife, paediatrician and anaesthetist. A glance at the clock as you call for help or start manoeuvres is helpful. Nominate someone to record the timing and sequence of events. The woman's buttocks should be at the edge of the bed and her back should be flat on the bed. Do not panic!
- ☐ **Evaluate** for **episiotomy**.
- ☐ **Legs**: Place the legs in McRoberts position, with full flexion and abduction of the hips – the thighs should touch the abdomen. This manoeuvre requires two assistants. Attempt delivery in this position for 60 seconds. If this fails, the woman should remain in this position while the next manoeuvre is performed.
- ☐ **Pressure**: Apply suprapubic pressure (to the anterior shoulder), directed sideways, towards the anterior surface of the fetal chest. Pressure should be applied continuously or by a rocking motion. Traction should be applied on the baby's head and neck, without lateral flexion of the neck.

If the above measures fail to deliver the shoulder (about 1 in 10 cases):

- ☐ **Enter** manoeuvres: start with the first of the following three manoeuvres and move to the next if unsuccessful in 60 seconds:
  - Insert the index and middle fingers behind the anterior shoulder and push it towards the baby's chest.
  - Woods' screw manoeuvre: apply pressure with two fingers behind the anterior shoulder and two fingers in front of the posterior shoulder.
  - Reverse Woods' screw: apply pressure with fingers behind the posterior shoulder.
- ☐ **Remove** the posterior arm. Deliver the posterior arm by following the humerus up to the elbow and flexing it. Grasp the wrist and sweep the arm across the chest until it is delivered.
- ☐ **Roll** the woman on to her hands and knees. Deliver the posterior arm by downward traction.

- If the above drill is not successful, and the baby is still alive, try either of the following:
  - o Replace the baby's head and proceed to CS. To push back the head, first convert it to the occipitoanterior position. Also, do this with the aid of a tocolytic.
  - o Perform a symphysiotomy.
- If the baby is dead, a cleidotomy may be performed.

After delivery

- ☐ Repair any perineal tear/episiotomy.
- ☐ Watch for PPH.
- ☐ Review the events with the woman and her partner.
- ☐ Complete an incident form.

Documentation

A local proforma is useful in capturing essential information. The following should be documented:

- ☐ the time of delivery of the head
- ☐ the direction the head was facing after restitution
- ☐ which shoulder was the anterior shoulder
- ☐ the manoeuvre(s) performed, including time and sequence
- ☐ the time of delivery of the body
- ☐ the staff in attendance and the time they arrived
- ☐ who else was present at delivery
- ☐ the condition of the baby
- ☐ any deficit in motion of the extremities and which extremity(ies)
- ☐ umbilical cord blood analysis
- ☐ any maternal injuries/complications

All babies with actual or suspected brachial plexus injury, whether or not there was recorded shoulder dystocia, should be examined by the neonatologist on duty once the diagnosis is made or suspected.

81 Cord prolapse

Cord prolapse is when the umbilical cord slips below the presenting part, with ruptured membranes.

It should always be excluded when spontaneous rupture of the membranes occurs and when amniotomy is performed.

Diagnosis may be suggested by sudden abnormalities on the CTG.

Risk factors

- breech presentation
- high head at onset of labour
- multiple pregnancy
- polyhydramnios
- preterm labour

Action plan

☐ Ring the emergency bell.

☐ Summon the registrar, anaesthetist and anaesthetic practitioner, and paediatrician.

☐ Push the presenting part above and away from the cord. Feel for pulsation, but avoid unnecessary handling.

☐ Place the woman in the knee/chest (all-fours) position. If an epidural is sited, place her in the left lateral position.

☐ Move the woman to theatre immediately.

☐ If cord pulsation is not palpable, use CTG and/or a scan to ascertain the status of the fetus.

☐ Explain to the woman and her partner what is happening.

☐ Deliver by CS unless:
  - the cervix is fully dilated and the presenting part is below the ischial spines (in which case use ventouse or forceps delivery), or
  - the baby is not alive.

☐ Measure umbilical cord pH.

☐ Discuss the event with the woman and her partner.

☐ Documentation: provide a chronological account of events and management.

If for any reason delivery is delayed, fill the bladder with 500 mL 0.9% saline. This relieves cord compression directly as well as indirectly (by inhibiting uterine contractions) – but do not forget to empty the bladder before proceeding with CS.

82 Anaphylaxis

Presentation

- itching
- flushing
- rash
- nausea
- vomiting
- breathlessness
- wheezing
- oedema
- tachycardia
- hypotension
- respiratory or cardiac collapse

Action plan

- ☐ Summon help.
- ☐ Discontinue/remove the offending agent.
- ☐ Assess airways, breathing and circulation, and commence basic life support if appropriate.
- ☐ Raise the feet to help restore BP.
- ☐ Administer oxygen by bag and mask.
- ☐ Give 0.5 mg adrenaline IM (i.e. 0.5 mL of 1 : 1000 injection). Repeat every 10 minutes until BP and pulse are normal or help arrives.
- ☐ Monitor vital signs and O_2 saturation.
- ☐ Insert a 14FG IV cannula.
- ☐ Give an IV infusion of Gelofusine or Haemaccel.
- ☐ Check arterial blood gases.
- ☐ Give chlorphenamine 10 mg IV, by slow infusion.
- ☐ Give hydrocortisone 100 mg IV immediately.
- ☐ Give aminophylline 250 mg IV over 20 minutes.
- ☐ Institute continuous electronic fetal monitoring, if the woman is prenatal.

83 Inverted uterus

Uterine inversion is when the fundus prolapses into the body of the uterus and beyond. It may occur spontaneously or as a result of mismanagement of the third stage of labour. It causes severe pain and may result in shock without evidence of bleeding. Haemorrhagic shock can occur if inversion has followed uterine atony.

Rapid colloid infusion may fail to improve the woman's condition, and care should be taken to avoid fluid overload.

Action plan

- ☐ If the woman is in shock, assess airways, breathing and circulation; summon help and commence basic life support if appropriate.
- ☐ Exclude submucous fibroid (the uterus will be palpable abdominally).
- ☐ Maintain IV access (18G cannula), and give Hartmann's solution.
- ☐ FBC.
- ☐ Cross-match 4 units of blood.
- ☐ Reduce the inverted uterus.
- ☐ Commence Syntocinon (oxytocin) infusion, 40 units in 500 mL 5% glucose following successful reduction.

Reduction of the inversion

Manual reduction

- **If the inversion occurs during delivery**, it may be possible to replace the uterus immediately with Entonox or IM pethidine. If effective epidural analgesia is already in place then this could be adequate. In all other circumstances, and **particularly if the woman is in shock**, reduction of an inverted uterus should be performed under a general anaesthetic.
- **If the placenta has not separated**, replace the uterus and commence Syntocinon infusion (40 units in 500 mL Hartmann's solution), and then perform manual removal of the placenta. Do not attempt to remove the placenta before replacing the uterus.

Hydrostatic reduction

- Exclude vaginal tear and rupture of the uterus before using this technique.
- Use *warm* saline (start with a 1 L bag) via a wide-bore giving set. The bag should be about 1 m above the patient (this gives a hydrostatic pressure of 100 cmH$_2$O). Do not use hypotonic fluid.
- The accoucheur covers the vaginal introitus with his/her hands, or with a 6 cm Silastic ventouse cup to provide a seal.
- **A general anaesthetic is not mandatory.**
- If the placenta has not separated, replace the uterus and commence Syntocinon infusion (40 units in 500 mL Hartmann's solution), and then perform manual removal of the placenta.
- Keep a record of the amounts of fluid infused into the vagina and released from it.

> **!** Do not attempt to remove the placenta before replacing the uterus, since doing so could increase haemorrhage, shock and intravasation of fluid.

Sometimes it will be necessary to administer a tocolytic. Rarely, it may be necessary to perform laparotomy and reduction from above.

Acute inversion may be complicated by pulmonary oedema from excessive IV fluids or, in cases of hydrostatic replacement, from fluid intravasation.

Discuss management of the third stage of labour in the next pregnancy.

84 Amniotic fluid embolism

This condition may occur suddenly in labour, at CS, or soon after delivery. The mortality rate is about 60–80%. Morbidity in survivors is high. Cardiovascular collapse and respiratory symptoms are the most common initial presentations.

A high index of suspicion could be life-saving. This rare condition must be suspected if there is:

- disorientation/agitation/delirium
- sudden shock (cardiovascular collapse)
- respiratory distress
- cyanosis
- fetal distress
- coma
- coagulopathy

If the above occur during labour or CS or within 30 minutes postpartum and there is no other explanation (i.e. the differential diagnoses have been excluded) then a clinical diagnosis of amniotic fluid embolism can be made.

Differential diagnoses

- PE
- myocardial infarction
- Mendelson's syndrome
- cerebrovascular accident
- total spinal
- septic shock
- substance abuse
- placental abruption
- eclampsia

Management

- [ ] Summon help.
- [ ] Commence basic life support.
- [ ] FBC.
- [ ] Obtain a coagulation profile: PT, APTT and fibrinogen.
- [ ] FDP/D-dimer.

- ☐ U/E.
- ☐ LFT.
- ☐ Obtain IV access; give IV fluids.
- ☐ Cross-match 4 units of blood.
- ☐ Chest X-ray.
- ☐ V/Q scan.
- ☐ ECG.
- ☐ Pulse oximetry.
- ☐ Set up automated BP monitoring.
- ☐ Insert a CVP line and arterial catheter.
- ☐ Insert a urinary catheter.
- ☐ CTG, if undelivered.
- ☐ Contact the consultant haematologist immediately – do not wait until coagulopathy is evident. Transfuse FFP, cryoprecipitate and platelets as advised by the haematologist. Liaise with the consultant anaesthetist.
- ☐ Transfer to ITU as soon as possible. If the woman is undelivered, an urgent CS should be performed before transfer.

Delivery should occur within 5 minutes of cardiac arrest, if there is no response to initial resuscitation (neonatal outcome is dependent on a short cardiac arrest-to-delivery interval).

Other aspects of management are as outlined in Chapter 85.

Amniotic fluid embolism register

Entry criteria

- acute hypotension or cardiac arrest
- acute hypoxia (dyspnoea, cyanosis or respiratory arrest)
- coagulopathy
- onset of all of the above during labour or CS, or within 30 minutes of delivery
- no other clinical condition or potential explanation for symptoms and signs

All cases meeting the above criteria, whether the patient survives or not, should be reported to Derek Tufnell, Bradford Royal Infirmary, Duckworth Lane, Bradford BD9 6RJ; Tel: 01274 364520.

85 Sudden maternal collapse

Possible causes

- PPH (possibly concealed in broad ligament or paravaginal haematoma)
- sepsis
- pneumothorax
- PE
- amniotic fluid embolism
- cardiac arrhythmia
- inverted uterus
- myocardial infarction
- left ventricular failure
- hypoglycaemia
- diabetic ketoacidosis
- cerebrovascular accident
- drug reaction
- anaphylaxis
- thyroid crisis
- uterine rupture
- peripartum cardiomyopathy
- ruptured aneurysm

Management

- [ ] Assess airways, breathing and circulation.
- [ ] Crash call (see p. xvii) and commence basic life support if appropriate; otherwise, turn the woman to the left lateral position.
- [ ] If CPR is required, ensure that pressure on the inferior vena cava by the pregnant uterus is relieved by means of a wedge under the woman's side.
- [ ] Examine for signs of vaginal bleeding, peritonitis and breathing difficulties.
- [ ] Consider intubation (by the anaesthetist, with cricoid pressure by the assistant), to reduce the risk of pulmonary aspiration.
- [ ] Give oxygen using bag and mask, 6 L/min
- [ ] Give an IV infusion of Haemaccel or Gelofusine.
- [ ] If the woman is in pain give IM pethidine 50–100 mg immediately.

Investigations

- ☐ FBC
- ☐ U/E
- ☐ LFT
- ☐ coagulation screen
- ☐ blood gases
- ☐ group and cross-match
- ☐ ECG
- ☐ portable chest X-ray

If the woman is diabetic, check her blood sugar with a glucometer and then give an infusion of 50 mL 50% glucose and insert a urinary catheter. Inform the on-call medical registrar.

If resuscitation has been unsuccessful after 5 minutes, proceed to CS – not only to save the baby but also to increase the mother's chances of survival.

86 Latex allergy

For the treatment of anaphylaxis, see Chapter 82.

Risk factors

- history of multiple surgical procedures
- history of atopy (hay fever, asthma, dermatitis or food allergy)
- previous anaphylactic episode of unknown cause, particularly if associated with surgery or dental treatment
- occupational exposure to latex

A latex-free pack for emergency use should always be available on the delivery suite.

Care of the woman allergic to latex

- Labour should be conducted in a latex-free room.
- Case notes, patient identification band and room door should carry warnings of latex allergy.
- Prepare a trolley with latex-free gloves, catheters, surgical tape, IV equipment and tourniquets for possible emergency use.
- Inform the anaesthetist.
- Management of IV drugs:
  - o draw up in latex-free syringes
  - o do not reconstitute or inject through rubber bungs.
- Beware of latex BP cuffs.
- Prepare a back-up theatre (to be latex-free) in case an emergency CS is required. The minimum dust-settling time is 2 hours.
- Drugs used to treat allergic reactions should be ready for use.

The following should not be used or left exposed in the care of a woman who is allergic to latex:

- latex gloves
- Foley catheter
- Entonox rubber tubing
- elasticated straps for CTG monitor
- rubber tourniquet
- sphygmomanometer tubing
- Elastoplast

- rubber mattress covers on theatre tables
- other rubber products

Theatre (elective or emergency procedure)

Only essential personnel should be in theatre.

Put up notices on theatre doors, marking the theatre as a latex-free room, and keep the doors shut.

SECTION 6
Stillbirths and congenital abnormalities

87 Checklist for fetal loss at 13–23 weeks

Parents

- ☐ The parents should be given the opportunity to see and hold the fetus.
- ☐ Has a minister of religion been requested?
- ☐ The parents should be offered a photograph.
- ☐ The parents should be informed about the choice of hospital or private funeral. An information leaflet should be provided.
- ☐ Postmortem examination should be discussed:
  - Has consent been given?
  - Has consent *not* been given?
- ☐ An appropriate bereavement pack should be provided.
- ☐ Has anti-D been given, if required?
- ☐ A follow-up appointment should be made.
- ☐ The woman should be seen by a doctor before discharge home.

Communication

- ☐ Arrange suppression of mail for parent education classes, antenatal clinic and other antenatal activities.
- ☐ The antenatal clinic should be informed of the fetal loss.
- ☐ The GP should be informed by telephone/fax and letter.

Forms/administration

- ☐ Complete all forms per local protocol.
- ☐ Complete the fetal loss register.
- ☐ Arrangements should be made for transport to the mortuary.
- ☐ Comply with local policy on sensitive disposal of fetal tissue.

88 Intrauterine fetal demise

Principles

- Be sure of the diagnosis before informing the woman.
- Keep the woman and her partner fully informed of what is happening.
- Show a caring attitude, but also give the woman and her partner the time and space that they require.
- The investigations performed will depend on whether there was an obvious cause of fetal loss.
- The issue of consent for postmortem examination is probably best brought up when discussing the cause of death.

Diagnosis (if not made before admission)

The first indication might be absence of fetal movement or inability to pick up fetal heart tones.

The obstetrician should perform an ultrasound scan. If fetal heart pulsation is not seen, the diagnosis should be confirmed by a practitioner who holds a formal qualification in ultrasound scanning. Inform the woman that fetal heart pulsation has not been seen but that a further scan is required and will be performed as soon as possible. Inform the consultant.

The senior obstetrician should discuss diagnosis and management with the woman. Decisions must be made regarding when and how to deliver the baby.

Administer mifepristone 200 mg orally, under supervision.

The GP, community midwife and health visitor should be informed, and antenatal appointments cancelled.

Action plan

Ideally, mifepristone should have been administered 36–48 hours before admission.

☐ Admit into a designated room.
☐ Discuss tests, including postmortem examination of the baby. Document which tests the woman/couple have consented to.
☐ Provide information booklets on funeral arrangements and postmortem examination.

☐ Ensure compliance with national policies and legislation; see Human Tissue Authority. *Code of Practice – Post Mortem Examination.* (Code 3: July 2006). Available at: www.hta.gov. uk/legislationpoliciesandcodesofpractice/codesofpractice.cfm.

☐ Document consent for tests. A standard form for 'Consent to a hospital post mortem examination on a baby or child' is available at: www.dh.gov.uk/en/Consultations/ Responsestoconsultations/DH_4080449.

☐ Induction of labour: see below.

☐ Investigations: see below.

☐ Consider antibiotic treatment.

☐ Discuss funeral arrangements – private or hospital burial – or disposal by the pathology laboratory.

☐ Offer counselling and provide details of support groups.

☐ If possible, avoid artificial rupture of membranes (risk of infection).

☐ Ask the parents if they wish to name the baby. Record the name in the notes.

☐ Examine the baby: wash, weigh, measure and label; check for abnormalities.

☐ Dress the baby (after examination, always keep the baby clothed).

☐ Parents should be allowed to see or hold the baby for as long as they wish.

☐ A photograph should be taken of the baby.

☐ A stillbirth certificate should be completed and signed.

☐ Prescribe medication to suppress lactation:
  - cabergoline 1 mg orally, single dose
  - bromocriptine 2.5 mg twice daily for 14 days is a less expensive option, but carries more risks; it should not be given to women with hypertension, coronary artery disease or any mental disorder.

☐ Arrange a follow-up appointment.

Investigations

Mother

Maternal blood tests

☐ FBC.

☐ HbA1c (glycated haemoglobin).

☐ blood group antibodies.

☐ Kleihauer test.

- ☐ Lupus anticoagulant.
- ☐ Anticardiolipin antibodies.
- ☐ Coagulation screen.
- ☐ TORCH screen (universal bottle, virology card): *Toxoplasma*, rubella, cytomegalovirus and hepatitis antibodies.
- ☐ Parvovirus B19 screen.
- ☐ Chromosome analysis, if not known.
- ☐ Any other clinically indicated blood test.

Urine

- ☐ Perform a drugs screen on a urine sample, if there is a suspicion of drug misuse.

Vagina

- ☐ Take a vaginal swab (during routine examination before inducing labour) for microscopy and culture.

Placenta

- ☐ Swab for culture.
- ☐ Send to pathology (for histology tests) in a bucket with formalin and a histology card.

Fetus

- ☐ Take a full-depth fetal skin biopsy (0.5 cm^3) from the axilla for cytogenetics/FISH:
  - Do not clean the skin before biopsy.
  - Skin biopsy culture usually fails in macerated stillbirth.
- ☐ Take a cord or cardiac blood sample (at least 0.5 mL into a 1–2 mL lithium heparin paediatric tube) for FBC, chromosome analysis and culture.
- ☐ Take swabs from nose, throat, ear and umbilicus for culture.
- ☐ Take photographs.
- ☐ Take an X-ray of the fetus.
- ☐ A postmortem should be offered (see Action plan above).

Induction of labour

Ensure that the fetal lie is longitudinal before induction of labour. If the lie is abnormal then the senior obstetrician should discuss version with the woman.

If fetal demise has occurred in mid-trimester, follow the algorithm described in Chapter 90.

If demise has occurred in the third trimester, assess the cervix and proceed as follows:

- **Cervix favourable**: perform amniotomy and commence a Syntocinon (oxytocin) infusion.
- **Cervix unfavourable for amniotomy but cervical score > 5**: insert prostaglandin E_2 (PGE_2, dinoprostone) gel 1 mg. Repeat 4 hours later if the cervix remains unfavourable for amniotomy.
- **Cervical score < 5, and no contraindications to gemeprost**: insert a gemeprost 1 mg pessary; repeat every 3 hours until labour is induced or amniotomy is feasible.
- **Cervical score < 5 and gemeprost contraindicated**: use dinoprostone gel 2 mg. If required, a further dose of dinoprostone gel 1 mg may be given 4 hours later.

> **!** Gemeprost should not be used in grandmultiparous women or in women with uterine scar.

If the cervix remains unfavourable for amniotomy despite two doses of dinoprostone gel, consider using extra-amniotic prostaglandin (see below).

If labour is not induced after five doses of gemeprost, allow 12–24 hours and then commence extra-amniotic prostaglandin as follows:

☐ One ampoule containing 5 mg of dinoprostone should be dissolved in 0.5 mL ethanol and 50 mL 0.9% saline. This gives a 100 µg/mL solution.

☐ Obtain a 12–14FG Foley catheter with a 30 mL balloon. Fill the dead space with 3 mL of the solution you have prepared.

☐ Under aseptic conditions, insert the catheter through the cervix and inflate the balloon.

☐ Start infusion at an initial rate of 1 mL/h, increasing to 2 mL/h if there is no uterine response after 4 hours.

☐ When the catheter falls out, amniotomy may be performed.

> **!** Note that dinoprostone potentiates the effect of Syntocinon on the uterus.

If labour is not induced despite the measures described above, further management will be determined by the consultant, based on the circumstances and preferences of the woman.

For twin delivery after 24 weeks when one twin is known to have died in utero before viability, the dead twin has to be registered as a stillbirth; it is assigned the gestational age of the live twin.

Support group

Sands (Stillbirth & Neonatal Death Charity)
   28 Portland Place
   London
   W1B 1LY

   Helpline: 020 7436 5881 (0930 to 1730, Monday to Friday)
   Office: 020 7436 7940 (1000 to 1700, Monday to Friday)
   Fax: 020 7436 3715
   Website: www.uk-sands.org

89 Mid-trimester termination of pregnancy for fetal abnormality

The principles of management are as outlined for intrauterine fetal demise (Chapter 88). Ensure that the statutory forms for termination of pregnancy have been completed.

Induction of labour

Follow the protocol described in Chapter 90.

Investigations

These will depend on the nature of the abnormality.

Prenatal diagnosis of chromosomal abnormality

- [ ] Take a full-depth fetal skin biopsy (0.5 cm³) for cytogenetics/FISH.
- [ ] Take a sample of cord (2–3 cm in length) and a sample of placental membrane from around the cord-insertion site.
- [ ] Take a cord or cardiac blood sample (at least 0.5 mL into a 1–2 mL lithium heparin paediatric tube).

Send solid specimens in dry pots – **do not use formalin.** If transport has to be delayed overnight, store at 4°C; **do not freeze**. Ensure that containers are labelled properly.

Ultrasound scan diagnosis of structural abnormality or external appearance suggestive of aneuploidy

The procedure is the same as outlined above.

Scan diagnosis of neural tube defect, with no other malformation or recurrences in family

Cytogenetic diagnosis is not routinely required in these cases.

Genetic examination of fetuses and samples

Only fetuses (and samples) aborted in the following circumstances should be sent to the laboratory:

- prenatal diagnosis of chromosomal abnormality
- scan diagnosis of structural abnormality (in the case of neural tube defects, those with other abnormalities or where there has been recurrence in the family)
- miscarriage where the baby has obvious malformations

Support group

Antenatal Results and Choices (ARC)
   73 Charlotte Street
   London
   W1T 4PN

   Helpline: 020 7631 0285 (1000 to 1730)
   Administration: 020 7631 0280 (1000 to 1730)
   Email: info@arc-uk.com
   Website: www.arc-uk.org

90 Protocol for medical termination of mid-trimester pregnancy

As part of the process of obtaining consent for this procedure, an information leaflet should be provided. The leaflet should include contact details.

Procedure

- [ ] The woman takes one tablet (200 mg) of mifepristone, witnessed by staff.
- [ ] She is observed for 1 hour. If vomiting occurs, give prochlorperazine 12.5 mg IM and repeat mifepristone.
- [ ] The woman is discharged home. The discharge information should include a contact telephone number.
- [ ] 36–48 hours later, the woman attends the ward and the procedure is explained again.
- [ ] Misoprostol 800 µg (or gemeprost 1 mg) is inserted into the posterior fornix.
- [ ] If the fetus/products have not been expelled, give oral misoprostol 400 µg every 4 hours (or gemeprost 1 mg pessary every 3 hours) up to a maximum of four doses.
- [ ] Analgesia should be given as required (co-codamol every 4 hours or diamorphine 5–10 mg IM every 4 hours).
- [ ] Record BP, pulse and temperature hourly.
- [ ] If the first course of treatment was successful and the woman is in a stable condition, discharge home, inform the GP, and confirm follow-up arrangements.
- [ ] If the first course of treatment was not successful, allow 12 hours from the last dose before commencing a second course of gemeprost pessaries, as above.

Contraindications

The use of mifepristone is contraindicated in the following cases:

- allergy to mifepristone
- chronic renal failure
- long-term corticosteroid therapy
- clotting disorders or anticoagulant therapy

- anaemia ([Hb] < 8.5 g/dL)
- smoker aged ≥35 years
- suspected ectopic pregnancy

The use of misoprostol or gemeprost is contraindicated in the following cases:

- allergy to prostaglandins
- severe asthma

Caution

Use mifepristone with caution in the following cases:

- asthma
- chronic obstructive airway disease
- cardiovascular disease
- renal failure
- liver failure
- prosthetic heart valves

Use misoprostol and gemeprost with caution in the following cases:

- cerebrovascular disease
- coronary artery disease
- severe peripheral vascular disease, including hypertension

Further reading for Part III

Caesarean section

Anorlu RI, Maholwans B, Hofmeyr GJ. Methods of delivering the placenta at caesarean section. *Cochrane Database Syst Rev* 2008; (3): CD004737.

Lucas DN, Yentis SM, Kinsella SM et al. Urgency of caesarean section: a new classification. *J R Soc Med* 2000; **93**: 346–50.

NHS Litigation Authority. Criterion 3.2.5. In: *Clinical Negligence Scheme for Trusts: Clinical Risk Management Standards for Maternity Services.* London: NHS Litigation Authority, 2002.

Small F, Hofmeyr GJ. Antibiotic prophylaxis for cesarean section. *Cochrane Database Syst Rev* 2002; (3): CD000933.

Thomas J, Paranjothy S; Royal College of Obstetricians and Gynaecologists Clinical Effectiveness Support Unit. *National Sentinel Caesarean Section Audit Report.* London: RCOG Press, 2001.

Recovery of obstetric patients

Association of Anaesthetists of Great Britain and Ireland. *Immediate Postanaesthetic Recovery.* London: AAGBI, September 2002. Available at: www.aagbi.org/ publications/guidelines.htm#i.

Association of Anaesthetists of Great Britain and Ireland and Obstetric Anaesthetists' Association. *OAA/AAGBI Guidelines for Obstetric Anaesthesia Services*, Revised Edition 2005. London: AAGBI and OAA, May 2005. Available at: www.aagbi.org/publications/guidelines/docs/obstetric05.pdf.

Fairfield MC, Bland D, Mushambi MC. Post-anaesthesia recovery care on the labour ward. *Int J Obstet Anesth* 1997; **6**: 153–5.

NHS Litigation Authority. Criterion 4.1.4. In: *Clinical Negligence Scheme for Trusts: Clinical Risk Management Standards for Maternity Services.* London: NHS Litigation Authority, 2002.

UK Health Departments. *Report on Confidential Enquiries into Maternal Deaths in the United Kingdom 1988–1990.* London: HMSO, 1994.

High-dependency care

Collis RE. Anaesthesia for caesarean section: general anaesthesia. In: Collis R, Plaat F, Urquhart J, eds. *Textbook of Obstetric Anaesthesia.* London: Greenwich Medical Media, 2002: 113–31.

Dhond GR, Ridley SA. Intensive and high dependency care of the obstetric patient. In: Collis R, Plaat F, Urquhart J, eds. *Textbook of Obstetric Anaesthesia.* London: Greenwich Medical Media, 2002: 235–50.

Failed intubation drill

Rahman K, Jenkins JG. Failed tracheal intubation in obstetrics: no more frequent but still managed badly. *Anaesthesia* 2005; **60**: 168–71.

Nair A, Alderson JD. Failed intubation drill in obstetrics. *Int J Obstet Anesth* 2006; **15**: 172–4.

Vasdev GM, Harrison BA, Keegan MT, Burkle CM. Management of the difficult and failed airway in obstetric anesthesia. *J Anesth* 2008; **22**: 38–48.

Instrumental delivery

Edozien LC. Towards safe practice in instrumental delivery. *Best Prac Res Clin Obstet Gynaecol* 2007; **21**: 639–55.

Edozien LC, Williams J, Chattopadhyay I, Hirsch PJ. Failed instrumental delivery: How safe is the use of a second instrument? *J Obstet Gynaecol* 1999; **19**: 460–2.

Johanson R, Menon V. Soft versus rigid vacuum extractor cups for assisted vaginal delivery. *Cochrane Database Syst Rev* 2000; (2): CD000446.

Murphy DJ, Liebling RE, Patel R et al. Cohort study of operative delivery in the second stage of labour and standard of obstetric care. *BJOG* 2003; **110**: 610–15.

Royal College of Obstetricians and Gynaecologists. *Operative Vaginal Delivery.* Clinical Green-top Guideline No. 26. London: Royal College of Obstetricians and Gynaecologists, October 2005. Available at: www.rcog.org.uk/files/rcog-corp/uploaded-files/GT26OperativeVaginalDelivery2005.pdf.

Sadan O, Ginath S, Gomel A et al. Vacuum application through a nonfully dilated cervix: a viable option. *Arch Gynecol Obstet* 2003; **268**: 281–3.

Trial of vaginal delivery after a previous caesarean section

American College of Obstetricians and Gynecologists. *Vaginal Birth after Previous Cesarean Delivery.* Practice Bulletin No. 5. Washington, DC: American College of Obstetricians and Gynecologists, 1999.

Chazotte C, Madden R, Cohen WR. Labor patterns in women with previous cesareans. *Obstet Gynecol* 1990; **75**: 350–5.

Khan KS, Rizvi A. The partograph in the management of labor following cesarean section. *Int J Gynaecol Obstet* 1995; **50**: 151–7.

Royal College of Obstetricians and Gynaecologists. *Birth after Previous Caesarean Birth.* Clinical Green-top Guideline No. 45. London: Royal College of Obstetricians and Gynaecologists, February 2007. Available at: www.rcog.org.uk/files/rcog-corp/uploaded-files/GT45BirthAfterPreviousCeasarean.pdf.

Induction of labour

National Institute for Health and Clinical Excellence. *Induction of Labour.* NICE Clinical Guideline 70. London: NICE, July 2008. Available at: http://guidance.nice.org.uk/CG70/Guidance/pdf/English.

Antenatal corticosteroid therapy

Roberts D, Dalziel SR. Antenatal corticosteroids for accelerating fetal lung maturation for women at risk of preterm birth. *Cochrane Database Syst Rev* 2006; (3): CD004454.

Royal College of Obstetricians and Gynaecologists. *Antenatal Corticosteroids to Prevent Respiratory Distress Syndrome*. Clinical Green-Top Guideline No. 7. London: Royal College of Obstetricians and Gynaecologists, February 2004. Available at: www.rcog.org.uk/files/rcog-corp/GT7AntenatalCorticosterodsamended.pdf.

Preterm prelabour rupture of membranes

Kenyon S, Boulvain M, Neilson J. Antibiotics for preterm rupture of membranes. *Cochrane Database Syst Rev* 2003; (2): CD001058.

Kenyon S, Taylor D, Tarnow-Mordi W. Broad spectrum antibiotics for preterm, prelabour rupture of fetal membranes: the ORACLE I randomised trial. *Lancet* 2001; **357**: 979–88.

Lamont RF. Recent evidence associated with the condition of preterm prelabour rupture of the membranes. *Curr Opin Obstet Gynecol* 2003; **15**: 91–9.

Waters TP, Mercer BM. The management of preterm premature rupture of the membranes near the limit of fetal viability. *Am J Obstet Gynecol*, 2009; **20**: 230–40.

Preterm uterine contractions

King J, Flenady V. Prophylactic antibiotics for inhibiting preterm labour with intact membranes. *Cochrane Database Syst Rev* 2002; (4): CD000246.

Morales WJ, Smith SG, Angel JA et al. Efficacy and safety of indomethacin versus ritodrine in the management of preterm labour: a randomized study. *Obstet Gynecol* 1989; **74**: 567–72.

Moutquin JM, Sherman D, Cohen HM et al. Double-blind, randomised, controlled trial of atosiban and ritodrine in the treatment of preterm labour: a multicenter effectiveness and safety study. *Am J Obstet Gynecol* 2000; **182**: 1191–9.

Papatsonis DN, van Geijn HP, Ader HJ et al. Nifedipine and ritodrine in the management of preterm labour: a randomised multicentre trial. *Obstet Gynecol* 1997; **90**: 230–4.

Royal College of Obstetricians and Gynaecologists. *Tocolytic Drugs for Women in Preterm Labour*. Clinical Green-top Guideline No. 1(B). London: Royal College of Obstetricians and Gynaecologists, October 2002. Available at: www.rcog.org.uk/files/rcog-corp/GT1BTocolyticDrug2002revised.pdf.

Worldwide Atosiban versus Beta-agonists Study Group. Effectiveness and safety of the oxytocin antagonist atosiban versus beta-adrenergic agonists in the treatment of preterm labour. *BJOG* 2001; **108**: 133–42.

Deliveries at the lower margin of viability

American Academy of Pediatrics Committee on Fetus and Newborn. American College of Obstetricians and Gynecologists Committee on Obstetric Practice. Perinatal care at the threshold of viability. *Pediatrics* 1995; **96**: 974–6.

British Association of Perinatal Medicine. *Fetuses and Newborn Infants at the Threshold of Viability: A Framework for Practice*. Memorandum. London: British Association of Perinatal Medicine, 1999.

Costeloe K, Hennessy E, Gibson AT et al. The EPICure study: outcomes to discharge from hospital for infants born at the threshold of viability. *Paediatrics* 2000; **106**: 659–71.

Rennie JM. Perinatal management at the lower margin of viability. *Arch Dis Child Fetal Neonatal Ed* 1996; **74**: F214–18.

Royal College of Obstetricians and Gynaecologists. *Late Termination of Pregnancy for Fetal Abnormality: A Consideration of the Law and Ethics*. London: Royal College of Obstetricians and Gynaecologists, 1998.

Multiple pregnancy

Baskett TF. *Essential Management of Obstetric Emergencies*, 3rd edn. Bristol: Clinical Press, 1999: 151–8.

Belfort MA. Intravenous nitroglycerin as a tocolytic agent for intrapartum external cephalic version. *S Afr Med J* 1993; **83**: 656–7.

Dufour PH, Vinatier S, Vanderstichele S et al. Intravenous nitroglycerin for intrapartum podalic version of the second twin in transverse lie. *Obstet Gynecol* 1998; **92**: 416–9.

Hofmeyr GJ, Drakeley AJ. Delivery of twins. *Baillieres Clin Obstet Gynaecol* 1998; **12**: 91–108.

Occipitoposterior position

Hunter S, Hofmeyr GJ, Kulier R. Hands and knees posture in late pregnancy or labour for fetal malposition (lateral or posterior). *Cochrane Database Syst Rev* 2007; (4): CD001063.

Shaffer BL, Cheng YW, Vargas JE et al. Manual rotation of the fetal occiput: predictors of success and delivery. *Am J Obstet Gynecol* 2006; **194**: e7–9.

Malpresentation

Singh S, Paterson-Brown S. Malpresentations in labour. *Curr Obstet Gynaecol* 2003; **13**: 300–6.

Breech presentation

Grant A, Glazener CM. Elective versus selective caesarean section for delivery of the small baby. *Cochrane Database Syst Rev*, 2001; (1): CD000078.

Hannah ME, Hannah WJ, Hewson SA et al; Term Breech Trial Collaborative Group. Planned caesarean section versus planned vaginal birth for breech presentation at term: a randomised multicentre trial. *Lancet* 2000; **356**: 1375–83.

Nwosu EC, Walkinshaw S, Chia P et al. Undiagnosed breech. *BJOG* 1993; **100**: 531–5.

Royal College of Obstetricians and Gynaecologists. *The Management of Breech Presentation.* Clinical Green-top Guideline No. 20b. London: Royal College of Obstetricians and Gynaecologists, December 2006. Available at: www.rcog.org. uk/files/rcog-corp/uploaded-files/GT20bManagement_ofBreechPresentation. pdf.

External cephalic version

Ben-Haroush A, Perri T, Bar J et al. Mode of delivery following successful external cephalic version. *Am J Perinatol* 2002; **19**: 355–60.

Bujold E, Marquette GP, Ferreira E et al. Sublingual nitroglycerin versus intravenous ritodrine as tocolytic for external cephalic version: a double-blinded randomized trial. *Am J Obstet Gynecol* 2003; **188**: 1454–7.

De Meeus JB, Ellia F, Magnin G. External cephalic version after previous caesarean section: a series of 38 cases. *Eur J Obstet Gynecol Reprod Biol* 1998; **81**: 65–8.

Ferguson JE 2nd, Dyson DC. Intrapartum external cephalic version. *Am J Obstet Gynecol* 1985; **152**: 297–8.

Hofmeyr GJ, Gyte GML. Interventions to help external cephalic version for breech presentation at term. *Cochrane Database Syst Rev* 2004; (1): CD000184.

Hofmeyr GJ, Kulier R. External cephalic version for breech presentation at term. *Cochrane Database Syst Rev* 1996; (1): CD000083.

Royal College of Obstetricians and Gynaecologists. *External Cephalic Version and Reducing the Incidence of Breech Presentation.* Clinical Green-top Guideline No. 20a. London: Royal College of Obstetricians and Gynaecologists, December 2006. Available at: www.rcog.org.uk/files/rcog-corp/uploaded-files/ GT20aExternalCephalica2006.pdf.

The woman with genital mutilation

Larsen U, Okonofua FE. Female circumcision and obstetric complications. *Int J Gynaecol Obstet* 2002; **77**: 255–65.

Royal College of Midwives. *Female Genital Mutilation (Female Circumcision).* Position Paper No. 21. London: Royal College of Midwives, 1998. Available at: www.rcm. org.uk/college/standards-and-practice/position-papers/?locale=en.

Royal College of Obstetricians and Gynaecologists. *Female Genital Mutilation and its Management.* Clinical Green-top Guideline No. 59 London: Royal College of Obstetricians and Gynaecologists, May 2009. Available at: www.rcog.org.uk/ files/rcog-corp/GreenTop53FemaleGenitalMutilation.pdf.

Perineal tear

Fernando R, Sultan AH, Kettle C et al. Radleys methods of repair for obstetric and sphincter injury. *Cochrane Database Syst Rev* 2006; (3): CD002866.

Keighley MRB, Radley S, Johanson R. Consensus on prevention and management of post-obstetric bowel incontinence and third degree tear. *Clin Risk* 2000; **6**: 231–7.

Kettle C, Johanson RB. Absorbable synthetic versus catgut suture material for perineal repair. *Cochrane Database Syst Rev* 1999; (4): CD000006.

Kettle C, Hills RK, Ismail KM. Continuous versus interrupted sutures for repair of episiotomy or second degree tears. *Cochrane Database Syst Rev* 2007; (4): CD000947.

Royal College of Obstetricians and Gynaecologists. *The Management of Third- and Fourth-Degree Perineal Tears*. Clinical Green-top Guideline No. 29. London: Royal College of Obstetricians and Gynaecologists, March 2007. Available at: http://www.rcog.org.uk/files/rcog-corp/uploaded-files/GT29ManagementThirdFourthDegreeTears2007.pdf.

Heart disease in labour

American College of Obstetricians and Gynaecologists. *Cardiac Disease in Pregnancy.* Technical Bulletin No. 168. Washington, DC: American College of Obstetricians and Gynaecologists, 1992.

Endocarditis Working Group of the British Society for Antimicrobial Chemotherapy. Antibiotic prophylaxis of infective endocarditis. *Lancet* 1990; **335**: 88–90.

Nelson-Piercy C. Cardiac disease. In: Lewis G, ed. *Saving Mothers' Lives: Reviewing maternal deaths to make motherhood safer – 2003–2005. The Seventh Report of the Confidential Enquiries into Maternal Deaths in the United Kingdom*. London: RCOG Press, 2007: 117–30.

Nelson-Piercy C. Heart disease. In: *Handbook of Obstetric Medicine*, 2nd edn. London: Martin Dunitz, 2002: 22–39.

Peripartum cardiomyopathy

Mehta NJ, Mehta RN, Khan IA. Peripartum cardiomyopathy: clinical and therapeutic aspects. *Angiology* 2001; **52**: 759–62.

Olagundoye VV, Seow Y, Ashworth MA. Peripartum cardiomyopathy: a forgotten diagnosis? *Hosp Med* 2003; **64**: 50–1.

Pearson GD, Veille JC, Rahimtoola S et al. Peripartum cardiomyopathy: National Heart, Lung and Blood Institute and Office of Rare Diseases (National Institutes of Health) workshop recommendations and review. *JAMA* 2000; **283**: 1183–8.

Pre-eclampsia

Brodie H, Malinow AM. Anaesthetic management of preeclampsia/eclampsia. *Int J Obstet Anesth* 1999; **8**: 110–24.

Chappell LC, Poulton L, Halligan A, Shennan AH. Lack of consistency in research papers over the definition of pre-eclampsia. *BJOG* 1999; **106**: 983–5.

Department of Health. *Why Mothers Die. Report of the Confidential Enquiries into Maternal Deaths in the UK, 1994–96*. London: The Stationery Office, 1998.

Duley L, Gülmezoglu AM, Henderson-Smart DT. Magnesium sulphate and other anticonvulsants for women with pre-eclampsia. *Cochrane Database Syst Rev* 2003; (2): CD000025.

Fay TN. *Labour Ward Rules*. London: BMJ Books, 2001: 114.

Hasan MA, Thomas TA, Prys-Roberts C. Comparison of automatic oscillometric arterial pressure measurement with conventional auscultatory measurement in the labour ward. *Br J Anaesth* 1993; **70**: 141–4.

Idama TO, Lindlow SW. Magnesium sulphate: a review of clinical pharmacology applied to obstetrics. *BJOG* 1998; **105**: 260–8.

Mabie WC, Gonzalez AR, Sibai BM, Amon E. A comparative trial of labetalol and hydralazine in the acute management of severe hypertension complicating pregnancy. *Obstet Gynecol* 1987; **70**: 328–33.

Magee LA, Cham C, Waterman EJ et al. Hydralazine for treatment of severe hypertension in pregnancy: meta-analysis. *BMJ* 2003; **327**: 955–64.

Mortl MG, Schneider MC. Key issues in assessing, managing and treating patients presenting with severe preeclampsia. *Int J Obstet Anesth* 2000; **9**: 39–44.

National High Blood Pressure Education Program: Working Group Report on High Blood Pressure in Pregnancy. *Am J Obstet Gynecol* 2000; **183**: S1–22.

Nielson JP. Hypertensive diseases of pregnancy. In: Lewis G, ed. *Why Mothers Die 1997–1999. The fifth report of the Confidential Enquiries into Maternal Deaths in the United Kingdom*. London: RCOG Press, 2001: 76–93.

Quinn M. Automated blood pressure measurement devices: a potential source of morbidity in preeclampsia? *Am J Obstet Gynecol* 1994; **170**: 1303–7.

Ramanathan J, Bennet K. Pre-eclampsia: fluids, drugs and anaesthetic management. *Anesthesiol Clin North Am* 2003; **21**: 145–63.

Reinders A, Cuckson AC, Jones CR et al. Validation of the Welch Allyn 'Vital Signs' blood pressure measurement device in pregnancy and pre-eclampsia. *BJOG* 2003; **110**: 134–8.

Robson SC, Pearson JF. Fluid restriction policies in preeclampsia are obsolete. *Int J Obstet Anesth* 1999; **8**: 49–55.

Waisman GD, Mayorga LM, Camera MI et al. Magnesium plus nifedipine: potentiation of hypotensive effect in preeclampsia? *Am J Obstet Gynecol* 1988; **159**: 308–9.

Witlin AG, Sibai BM. Magnesium sulfate therapy in preeclampsia and eclampsia. *Obstet Gynecol* 1998; **92**: 883–9.

Eclampsia

Duley L, Carroli G, Belizan J et al. Which anticonvulsant for women with eclampsia – evidence from the collaborative eclampsia trial. *Lancet* 1995; **345**: 1455–63.

Duley L, Henderson-Smart D. Magnesium sulphate versus diazepam for eclampsia. *Cochrane Database Syst Rev* 2003; (4): CD000127.

Royal College of Obstetricians and Gynaecologists. *The Management of Severe Pre-eclampsia/Eclampsia*. Clinical Green-top Guideline No. 10(A). London: Royal College of Obstetricians and Gynaecologists, March 2006. Available at: www.rcog.org.uk/files/rcog-corp/uploaded-files/GT10aManagementPreeclampsia2006.pdf.

Diabetes mellitus

Chauhan SP, Perry KG Jr. Management of diabetic ketoacidosis in the obstetric patient. *Obstet Gynecol Clin North Am* 1995; **22**: 143–55.

Diabetes UK. *Recommendations for the Management of Pregnant Women with Diabetes (Including Gestational Diabetes)*. London: Diabetes UK, 2003.

Hadden DR, McCance DR. Advances in management of type 1 diabetes and pregnancy. *Curr Opin Obstet Gynecol* 1999; **11**: 557–62.

Lean ME, Pearson DW, Sutherland HW. Insulin management during labour and delivery in mothers with diabetes. *Diabet Med* 1990; **7**: 162–4.

Asthma (acute exacerbation in labour)

British Thoracic Society and Scottish Intercollegiate Guidelines Network. *British Guidelines on the Management of Asthma. A national clinical guideline*. London and Edinburgh: BTS and SIGN, 2009.

National Asthma Education and Prevention Program. *Working Group Report on Managing Asthma during Pregnancy: Recommendations for Pharmacologic Treatment – Update 2004*. US Department of Health and Human Services. National Institutes of Health, National Heart, Lung, and Blood Institute. NIH Publication No. 05-5236, March 2005.

Epilepsy

Katz JM, Devinsky O. Primary generalized epilepsy: a risk factor for seizures in labor and delivery? *Seizure* 2003; **12**: 217–19.

Pennell PB. Pregnancy in the woman with epilepsy: maternal and fetal outcomes. *Semin Neurol* 2002; **22**: 299–308.

Royal College of Midwives. *The Care of Women with Epilepsy – Guidelines for Midwives*. London: Royal College of Midwives, 1997.

Scottish Obstetric Guidelines and Audit Project. *The Management of Pregnancy in Women with Epilepsy. A Clinical Practice Guideline for Professionals Involved in Maternity Care*. Aberdeen: Scottish Programme for Clinical Effectiveness in Reproductive Health, 1997.

Systemic lupus erythematosus

Buchanan NMM, Khamashta MA, Kerslake S et al. Practical management of pregnancy in systemic lupus erythematosus. *Fet Mat Med Rev* 1993; **5**: 223–30.

Georgiou PE, Politi EN, Katsimbri P et al. Outcome of lupus pregnancy: a controlled study. *Rheumatology (Oxford)* 2000; **39**: 1014–19.

Mascola MA, Repke JT. Obstetric management of the high-risk lupus pregnancy. *Rheum Dis Clin North Am* 1997; **23**: 119–32.

Mok CC, Wong RW. Pregnancy in systemic lupus erythematosus. *Postgrad Med J* 2001; **77**: 157–65.

Other connective tissue disorders

Abouleish E. Obstetric anaesthesia and Ehlers–Danlos syndrome. *Br J Anaesth* 1980; **52**: 1283–6.

Lipscomb KJ, Clayton-Smith J, Clarke B et al. Outcome of pregnancy in women with Marfan syndrome. *BJOG* 1997; **104**: 201–4.

Roop KA, Brost BC. Abnormal presentation in labor and fetal growth of affected infants with type III Ehlers–Danlos syndrome. *Am J Obstet Gynecol* 1999; **181**: 752–3.

Stone S, Nelson-Piercy C. Connective tissue diseases in pregnancy. *Contemp Clin Gynecol Obstet* 2001; **1**: 69–81.

The rhesus-negative woman

Crowther C, Middleton P. Anti-D administration after childbirth for preventing Rhesus alloimmmunisation. *Cochrane Database Syst Rev* 2000; (2): CD000021.

National Institute for Health and Clinical Excellence. *Routine Antenatal Anti-D Prophylaxis for Women who are Rhesus D Negative.* NICE Technology Appraisal Guidance 156. London: NICE, August 2008. Available at: www.nice.org.uk/nicemedia/pdf/TA156Guidance.pdf.

Royal College of Obstetricians and Gynaecologists. *Use of Anti-D Immunoglobulin for Rh Prophylaxis.* Clinical Green-top Guideline No. 22. London: Royal College of Obstetricians and Gynaecologists, 2002. Available at: www.rcog.org.uk/womens-health/clinical-guidance/use-anti-d-immunoglobulin-rh-prophylaxis-green-top-22.

Thromboembolism prophylaxis

Confidential Enquiry into Maternal and Child Health. Summary of the key recommendations of the Royal College of Obstetricians and Gynaecologists (RCOG) guidelines for thromboprophylaxis in pregnancy, labour and after vaginal delivery and caesarean section. In Lewis G, ed. *Saving Mothers' Lives: Reviewing maternal deaths to make motherhood safer – 2003–2005. The Seventh Report of the Confidential Enquiries into Maternal Deaths in the United Kingdom.* London: 2007: 67–9.

Nelson-Piercy C. Obstetric thromboprophylaxis. *Br J Hosp Med* 1996; **55**: 404–8.

Acute venous thromboembolism and pulmonary embolism

Checketts MR, Wildsmith JA. Central nerve block and thromboprophylaxis – Is there a problem? *Br J Anaesth* 1999; **82**: 164–7.

Greer I. Treatment of venous thromboembolism in pregnancy. *Reprod Vasc Med* 2001; **1**: 114–19.

Horlocker TT, Wedel DJ. Spinal and epidural blockade and peri-operative low molecular weight heparin: smooth sailing on the Titanic. *Anesth Analg* 1998; **86**: 1153–6.

Royal College of Obstetricians and Gynaecologists. *Thromboembolic Disease in Pregnancy and the Puerperium: Acute Management.* Clinical Green-Top Guideline No. 28. London: Royal College of Obstetricians and Gynaecologists, February 2007. Available at: www.rcog.org.uk/files/rcog-corp/uploaded-files/GT28ThromboembolicDisease2007.pdf.

Major haemoglobinopathy

Danzer BI, Birnbach DJ, Thys DM. Anaesthesia for the parturient with sickle cell disease. *J Clin Anaesth* 1996; **8**: 598–602.

Howard RJ. Management of sickling conditions in pregnancy. *Br J Hosp Med* 1996; **56**: 7–10.

Howard RJ, Tuck SM. Sickle cell disease and pregnancy. *Curr Obstet Gynaecol* 1995; **5**; 36–40.

Rust OA, Perry KG Jr. Pregnancy complicated by sickle haemoglobinopathy. *Clin Obstet Gynaecol* 1995; **38**: 472–84.

Inherited coagulation disorders: haemophilia and von Willebrand's disease

Chi C, Kulkavni A, Lee CA et al. The obstetric experience of women with Factor XI deficiency. *Acta Obstet Gynecol Scand* 2009; **88**: 1095–100.

Conti M, Mari D, Conti E et al. Pregnancy in women with different types of von Willebrand disease. *Obstet Gynecol* 1986; **68**: 282–5.

Kadir RA. Women and inherited bleeding disorders: pregnancy and delivery. *Semin Hematol* 1999; **36**(3 suppl 4): 28–35.

Kadir RA, Economides DL, Braithwaite J et al. The obstetric experience of carriers of haemophilia. *BJOG* 1997; **104**: 803–10.

Kadir RA, Lee CA, Sabin CA et al. Pregnancy in women with von Willebrand's disease or factor XI deficiency. *BJOG* 1998; **105**: 314–21.

Walker ID, Walker JJ, Colvin BT et al. Investigation and management of haemorrhagic disorders in pregnancy. Haemostasis and Thrombosis Task Force. *J Clin Pathol* 1994; **47**: 100–8.

Immune thrombocytopenic purpura

Letsky EA. Haemostasis and epidural anaesthesia. *Int J Obstet Anaesth* 1991; **1**: 51–4.

Letsky EA, Greaves M. Guidelines on the investigation and management of thrombocytopenia in pregnancy and neonatal alloimmune thrombocytopenia. *Br J Haematol* 1996; **95**: 21–6.

Thrombophilia

Walker ID. Inherited coagulation disorders and thrombophilia in pregnancy. In: Bonnar J, ed. *Recent Advances in Obstetrics and Gynaecology*, No. 20. Edinburgh: Churchill Livingstone, 1998.

Walker ID. Management of thrombophilia in pregnancy. *Blood Rev* 1991; **5**: 227–33.

Gestational thrombocytopenia

Aster RH. 'Gestational' thrombocytopenia: a plea for conservative management. *N Engl J Med* 1990; **323**: 264–6.

Major placenta praevia

Penna LK, Pearce JM. Placenta praevia. In: Studd J, ed. *Progress in Obstetrics and Gynaecology*, Vol 11. Edinburgh: Churchill Livingstone, 1994.

Royal College of Obstetricians and Gynaecologists. *Placenta Praevia and Placenta Praevia Accreta: Diagnosis and Management.* Clinical Green-top Guideline No. 27. London: Royal College of Obstetricians and Gynaecologists, October 2005. Available at: www.rcog.org.uk/files/rcog-corp/uploaded-files/GT27PlacentaPreviaAccreta2005.pdf.

Sunna E, Ziadeh S. Transvaginal and transabdominal ultrasound for the diagnosis of placenta praevia. *J Obstet Gynaecol* 1999; **19**: 152–4.

Retained placenta

Carroli G, Bergel E. Umbilical vein injection for management of retained placenta. *Cochrane Database Syst Rev* 2001; (2): CD001337.

Postpartum haemorrhage

American Academy of Family Physicians. *Advanced Life Support in Obstetrics (ALSO) Course Syllabus*, 4th edn. Kansas: American Academy of Family Physicians, 2000.

Anorlu RI, Maholwana B, Hofmeyr GJ. Methods of delivering the placenta at caesarean section. *Cochrane Database Syst Rev* 2008; (3): CD004737.

Drife J. Management of primary postpartum haemorrhage. *BJOG* 1997; **104**: 275–7.

Hall M. Haemorrhage. In: Lewis G, ed. *Why Mothers Die 1997–1999. The Confidential Enquiries into Maternal Deaths in the United Kingdom.* London: RCOG Press, 2001: 94–103.

Disseminated intravascular coagulopathy

Thachil J, Toh CH. Disseminated intravascular coagulation in obstetric disorders and its acute haematological management. *Blood Rev* 2009; **23**: 167–76.

Delivery of the woman at known risk of haemorrhage

Hall MH. Haemorrhage. In: Lewis G, ed. *Why Mothers Die 1997–1999. The Confidential Enquiries into Maternal Deaths in the United Kingdom.* London: RCOG Press, 2001: 94–103.

Management of the woman who declines blood transfusion

Bonakdar MI, Eckhous AW, Backer BJ et al. Major gynaecologic and obstetric surgery in Jehovah's Witnesses. *Obstet Gynaecol* 1982; **60**: 587–90.

Buscuttil D, Copplestone A. Management of blood loss in Jehovah's Witness. *BMJ* 1995; **311**: 1115–16.

Confidential Enquiry into Maternal and Child Health. Guidelines for the management and treatment of obstetric haemorrhage in women who decline blood transfusion. In: Lewis G, ed. *Why Mothers Die 2000–2002. The Sixth Report of the Confidential Enquiries into Maternal Deaths in the United Kingdom.* London: RCOG Press, 2004: 94–5.

Mann CM, Votto J, Kambe J, McNamee MJ. Management of the severely anaemic patient who refuses transfusion: lessons learned during the care of a Jehovah's Witness. *Ann Intern Med* 1992; **177**: 1042–8.

Reid MF, Nohn R, Birks RJS. Eclampsia and haemorrhage in a Jehovah's Witness. *Anaesthesia* 1986; **41**: 324–5.

Thomas JM. The worldwide need for education in nonblood management in obstetrics and gynaecology. *J Soc Obstet Gynaecol Can* 1994; **16**: 1483–7.

Prophylactic antibiotics

British Society for Antimicrobial Chemotherapy. Endocarditis Working Party. Antibiotic prophylaxis of infective endocarditis. *Lancet* 1997; **350**: 1100.

Hopkins L, Smaill F. Antibiotic prophylaxis regimens and drugs for cesarean section. *Cochrane Database Syst Rev* 1999; (2): CD001136.

PHLS Group B Streptococcus Working Group. *Interim 'Best Practice' Recommendations for the Prevention of Neonatal Group B Streptococcal Infection in the UK.* London: Central Public Health Laboratory, 2000.

Intrapartum pyrexia

Harper A. Genital tract sepsis. In: Lewis G, ed. *Saving Mothers' Lives: Reviewing maternal deaths to make motherhood safer – 2003–2005. The Seventh Report of the Confidential Enquiries into Maternal Deaths in the United Kingdom.* London: RCOG Press, 2007: 97–106.

Intrapartum antibiotic prophylaxis for group B streptococci

American Academy of Pediatrics. Revised guidelines for prevention of early-onset group B streptococcal disease. *Pediatrics* 1997; **99**: 489–96.

Centers for Disease Control. Prevention of perinatal group B streptococcal disease: a public health perspective. *Morb Mortal Wkly Rep* 1996; **45**(RR-7): 1–20.

PHLS Group B Streptococcus Working Group. *Interim 'Best Practice' Recommendations for the Prevention of Neonatal Group B Streptococcal Infection in the UK.* London: Central Public Health Laboratory, 2000.

Royal College of Obstetricians and Gynaecologists. *Prevention of Early Onset Neonatal Group B Streptococcal Disease.* Clinical Green-top Guideline No. 36. London: Royal College of Obstetricians and Gynaecologists, November 2003. Available at: www.rcog.org.uk/files/rcog-corp/uploaded-files/GT36GroupBStrep2003.pdf.

Smaill F. Intrapartum antibiotics for group B streptococcal colonisation. *Cochrane Database Syst Rev* 1996: (1): CD000115.

Genital herpes

McLean A, Regan L, Carrington D. *Infection and Pregnancy. Report of an RCOG Study Group.* London: RCOG Press, 2001.

Royal College of Obstetricians and Gynaecologists. *Management of Genital Herpes in Pregnancy.* Clinical Green-top Guideline No. 30. London: Royal College of Obstetricians and Gynaecologists, September 2007. Available at: www.rcog.org.uk/files/rcog-corp/uploaded-files/GT30GenitalHerpes2007.pdf.

Smith JR, Cowan FM, Munday P. The management of herpes simplex virus infections in pregnancy. *BJOG* 1998; **105**: 255–60.

Human immunodeficiency virus

British HIV Association. Guidelines for the management of HIV infection in pregnant women and the prevention of mother-to-child transmission. *HIV Med* 2001; **2**: 314–34.

Irish Infection Society. National guidelines for the active management of HIV in pregnancy. *Ir Med J* 2001; **94**: 137–40.

Kuczkowski KM. Human immunodeficiency virus in the parturient. *J Clin Anesth* 2003; **15**: 224–33.

Minkoff H. Human immunodeficiency virus infection in pregnancy. *Obstet Gynecol* 2003; **101**: 797–810.

Public Health Service Task Force Perinatal HIV Guidelines Working Group. Summary of the updated recommendation from the Public Health Service Task Force to reduce perinatal human immunodeficiency virus-1 transmission in the United States. *Obstet Gynaecol* 2002; **99**: 1117–26.

Royal College of Midwives. *HIV and AIDS.* Position Paper 16a. London: Royal College of Midwives, October 1998. Available at: www.rcm.org.uk/college/standards-and-practice/position-papers/?locale=en.

Cervical tear and paravaginal haematoma

Ridgway LE. Puerperal emergency: vaginal and vulval haematoma. *Obstet Gynecol Clin North Am* 1995; **22**: 275–82.

Sheikh GN. Perinatal genital haematomas. *Obstet Gynecol* 1971: **38**: 571–5.

Rupture of the uterus

Clements RV. Operative obstetrics. In: Clements RV, ed. *Risk Management and Litigation in Obstetrics and Gynaecology.* London: Royal Society of Medicine Press, 2001: 238–40.

Shoulder dystocia

American Academy of Family Physicians. *Advanced Life Support in Obstetrics (ALSO) Course Syllabus*, 4th edn. Kansas: American Academy of Family Physicians, 2000.

Johnstone FD, Myerscough PR. Shoulder dystocia. *BJOG* 1998; **105**: 811–15.

Chauhan SP, Gherman R, Hendrix NW et al. Shoulder dystocia: Comparison of the ACOG practice bulletin with another national guidelines. *Am J Perinatal* 2009; **27**: 129–36.

Anaphylaxis

Anaphylaxis. In: *British National Formulary.* London: BMJ Group/RPS Publishing, updated twice-yearly. Available at: www.bnf.org/bnf/bnf/current/201198.htm.

Inverted uterus

Irani S, Jordan J. Management of uterine inversion. *Curr Obstet Gynaecol* 1997; **7**: 232–5.

Johnson NP, Bishop E, Buist R. Hydrostatic replacement of acute inversion of the uterus can cause acute pulmonary oedema by intrauterine fluid intravasation. *J Obstet Gynaecol* 1999; **19**: 544–5.

Ogueh O, Ayida G. Acute uterine inversion: a new technique of hydrostatic replacement. *BJOG* 1997; **104**: 951–2.

Rachagan SP, Sivanesratnam V, Kok KP, Raman S. Acute puerperal inversion of the uterus – an obstetric emergency. *Aust NZ J Obstet Gynaecol* 1988; **28**: 29–32.

Amniotic fluid embolism

Clark SL, Hankins GDV, Dudley DA et al. Amniotic fluid embolism: analysis of the national registry. *Am J Obstet Gynecol* 1995; **172**: 1158–69.

Howell P, Amniotic fluid embolism. In: Collis R, Plaat F, Urquhart J, eds. *Textbook of Obstetric Anaesthesia.* London: Greenwich Medical Media, 2002: 263–89.

Sudden maternal collapse

Advanced Life Support Working Group of the European Resuscitation Council. The 1998 European Resuscitation Council guidelines for adult advanced life support. *BMJ* 1998; **316**: 1863–9.

Hayashi RH. Obstetric collapse. In: Kean L, Baker PN, Edelstone DI, eds. *Best Practice in Labour Ward Management.* Edinburgh: WB Saunders, 2000.

Latex allergy

Adeley J, Rowland A. Managing the risk of latex allergy in healthcare workers and patients. *Clin Risk* 1999; **5**: 129–31.

Diaz T, Martinez T, Antepara I et al. Latex allergy as a risk during delivery. *BJOG* 1996; **103**: 173–5.

Eckhout GV Jr, Ayad S. Anaphylaxis due to airborne exposure to latex in a primigravida. *Anesthesiology* 2001; **4**: 1034–5.

Santos R, Hernandez-Ayup S, Galache P et al. Severe latex allergy after a vaginal examination during labour: a case report. *Am J Obstet Gynecol* 1997; **177**: 1543–4.

Shingai Y, Nakagawa K, Kato T et al. Severe allergy in a pregnant woman after vaginal examination with a latex glove. *Gynecol Obstet Invest* 2002; **54**: 183–4.

Mid-trimester termination of pregnancy for fetal abnormality

Royal College of Obstetricians and Gynaecologists. *Termination of Pregnancy for Fetal Abnormality in England, Wales and Scotland.* London: RCOG, 1996.

APPENDICES

Appendix A: Guidance for obtaining consent to treatment

Every adult woman of sound mind has a right to determine what can be done with her own body. She has an absolute right to refuse to consent to treatment for any reason, rational or irrational, or for no reason at all, even where the decision may lead to her own death. A healthcare provider who treats a woman without her consent could be liable in negligence or in the crime of battery. In the context of the guidance below, 'treatment' includes diagnostic procedures.

Good practice requires the provider to ensure that the patient understands what is proposed and consents to it, before proceeding with treatment or investigation. Where some form of consent has been given, it is important not to exceed the consent given or to carry out a procedure unrelated to the consent.

Who gives consent?

No one can legally give consent on behalf of an adult of sound mind. A spouse or other relative may not give consent or withhold consent if the woman is competent.

How valid is a consent?

The following are necessary for a consent to be valid:

- The patient must have the mental capacity to make the decision.
- The patient must make the decision without undue influence.
- The patient must be given sufficient information about the treatment.

If there is any doubt about the competence of a patient then the consultant should be informed. Guidance can be obtained from *Assessment of Mental Capacity: Guidance for Doctors and Lawyers* (see 'Further reading' at the end of this appendix). In some cases, it might be necessary to seek a court declaration.

Consent should not be obtained under duress. Where there is a recognized undue influence, this should be reported to the supervising consultant or senior midwife.

The professional obtaining consent should declare any potential conflict of interest.

The patient should be given sufficient time to consider the information given. For elective procedures, a reasonable interval should elapse between obtaining consent and performing treatment.

How much information should be given?

This is generally a matter of clinical judgement, depending on individual needs and the complexity of treatment; but enough information should be given to ensure that the patient understands:

- the nature of the treatment
- the benefits of the treatment
- the consequences of the treatment and of refusal of treatment
- any substantial risk of the treatment

Where there are alternatives, these should be discussed and reasons should be given for recommending a particular option. Oral information should be supplemented with information leaflets wherever possible. The use of such leaflets should be recorded.

Who should obtain consent?

To ensure that the patient is fully informed, it is important that her consent be obtained by the person who will provide the treatment. However, this task may be delegated to any professional who:

- is suitably trained and competent
- has sufficient knowledge of the proposed treatment
- understands the risks involved
- has access to an appropriate support person

The person providing the treatment remains responsible for ensuring that a meaningful consent has been given.

When is a written consent required?

Express (as opposed to implied) consent may be oral or written. An oral consent is as valid as a written consent, but written consent provides documentary evidence that a discussion took place.

Where oral consent has been obtained, it should be documented in the notes. This should be sufficient for most non-invasive procedures.

Written consent should be obtained for any procedure or treatment carrying any substantial risk or substantial side-effect.

> ! Shorthand and abbreviations should not be used and alterations to the consent form should be avoided.

Special cases

- A minor under 16 can give consent if she is Fraser (Gillick) competent.
- An official link worker should be used if the patient does not speak English.
- Arrangements must be made for patients with hearing or speech disabilities.

Procedures for which written consent should be obtained

- All procedures performed in theatre under local or general anaesthesia.
- Amniocentesis.
- Medical termination of pregnancy.

Procedures for which verbal consent should be obtained and documented

- Blood transfusion.
- Induction of labour.
- Vaginal examination in labour.
- Rectal examination.
- Vaginal examination by a medical student.
- Amniotomy, artificial rupture of fetal membranes (ARM).
- Breech vaginal delivery.
- Instrumental delivery.
- Administration of vitamin K injection to a baby.
- ECV.
- Fetal scalp blood sampling.
- Epidural analgesia.

- Administration of enema/suppository.
- Application of a fetal scalp electrode.
- Administration of anti-D immunoglobulin.
- Syntometrine (ergometrine with oxytocin) injection.
- Episiotomy.
- Repair of episiotomy.

Further reading

British Medical Association and The Law Society. *Assessment of Mental Capacity: Guidance for Doctors and Lawyers*, 2nd. edn, London: BMJ Books, 2004.

Department of Health. *Reference Guide to Consent for Examination or Treatment.* London: Department of Health, April 2001. Available at: www.dh.gov.uk/en/ Publicationsandstatistics/Publications/PublicationsPolicyAndGuidance/DH_ 4006757.

General Medical Council. *Consent: Patients and Doctors Making Decisions Together.* London: General Medical Council, 2008. Available at: www.gmc-uk.org/ guidance/ethical_guidance/consent_guidance/index.asp.

Royal College of Obstetrics and Gynaecologists. *Obtaining Valid Consent. Clinical Governance Advice, No. 6.* London: Royal College of Obstetrics and Gynacologists, 2008. Available at : www.rcog.org.uk/files/rcog-corp/uploaded-files/CGAObtainingValidConsent122008.pdf.

Appendix B: Standards for administering blood transfusion

Background

Despite improvements in the safety of blood transfusion, errors still occur, sometimes resulting in fatality. Errors commonly arise from incorrect labelling of a blood sample, laboratory mistakes or administering the blood product to the wrong patient. Most of the errors occur not in emergency intraoperative situations, but on the wards.

> There were 76 cases (of inappropriate and unnecessary transfusions) reported, with the largest group involving patients transfused on the basis of an erroneous laboratory value resulting from sampling, transcription or communication errors. A further significant category includes cases in which transfusion was given as a result of poor knowledge and decision making. There were two fatalities in this group: one from a massive over-transfusion, and one from under-transfusion, as well as one case of major morbidity. Attainment of appropriate knowledge and experience in transfusion medicine for clinical staff remains a major issue for medical educators.
>
> Serious Hazards in Transfusion (SHOT) Annual Report, 2008.

The single most important error resulting in mistransfusion is failure of the bedside checking procedure immediately before administering the transfusion.

This guidance is written to inform the training and practice of staff on the maternity unit, with a view to preventing errors in the administration of blood products. It should be read in conjunction with the hospital policy on blood transfusion.

Indications and techniques of blood transfusion are outside the scope of this appendix.

Obtaining consent

Except in emergencies or unconscious patients, the purpose, benefits and risks of blood transfusion should be explained to the patient. The alternatives to transfusion and the implications of declining a transfusion should also be discussed.

This discussion, and the patient's verbal consent to blood transfusion, should be documented.

The patient should be given the information leaflet *Your Questions about Blood Transfusion Answered* (see 'Further reading' at the end of this appendix).

Collecting a specimen for group-and-save/cross-match

The labels and cards must be completed *at the patient's bedside*, with the case notes available for reference.

Do not use pre-labelled bottles. First obtain the blood specimen, and then label the bottles at the bedside.

The blood specimen should not be obtained from an arm being used for infusion of IV fluids.

When the doctor signs the request form, he or she is confirming that the sample is identified correctly.

Previous transfusion records should be consulted.

An IV cannula should be sited before the cross-matched blood is sent for.

Checking procedure for blood transfusion

Ensure that *this* blood product is for *this* patient:

- Before transfusion, the labelling on the blood product must be checked against specific patient-identification details. This check must be carried out by two members of staff, one of whom must be a registered nurse or midwife.
- Read the wristband and check that this corresponds to the label on the blood product. Errors with wristbands may occur, so, if the patient is conscious, ask her to state her forename, family name and date of birth.
- If there are any discrepancies in spelling or identification number, transfusion should be withheld and the blood transfusion department contacted immediately.
- Check the records of any previous blood grouping against the current report.
- There are two labels on the blood product bag, indicating:
  - name of patient
  - hospital number
  - patient's blood group
  - donor unit number
  - compatibility type

○ donor's blood group
○ date and time of transfusion

These details must be checked against the form sent with the blood from the blood bank, and signed. One label must be removed and put in the patient's records.

- The final bedside check provides an important opportunity to detect errors that may have been made earlier in the process of requesting blood.

> **!** The inappropriate use of the compatibility form for the bedside checking of blood components and patient identification resulted in 18 cases of wrong blood administration in 2008.
>
> Serious Hazards in Transfusion (SHOT) Annual Report, 2008.

Documentation

The following should be entered in the case notes:

- consent (verbal will suffice)
- details of all blood products transfused (as above)
- the times at which transfusion commenced and ended
- observations, including pulse rate and temperature
- any transfusion reactions

Errors should be documented and reported as prescribed in the hospital's policy on significant event reporting.

Observation should continue for 24 hours after blood transfusion.

Further reading

McClelland DBL, ed. *Handbook of Transfusion Medicine*, 3rd edn. London: The Stationery Office, 2001.

National Blood Service. *Your Questions about Blood Transfusion Answered* (Information Leaflet). London: National Blood Service, 2001.

Serious Hazards of Transfusion (SHOT). *Annual Reports 2008*. Manchester: SHOT Steering Group. Available at: www.shotuk.org/SHOT%20report%202008.pdf

Szama K. 355 reports of transfusion-associated deaths. *Transfusion* 1990; **30**: 583.

Szama K. Practical issues in informed consent for blood transfusion. *Am J Clin Pathol* 1997; **107**: S72–4.

Williams FG. Consent for transfusion. A duty of care. *BMJ* 1997; **315**: 380–1.

INDEX